Transanal Stapling Techniques for Anorectal Prolapse

Transanal Stapling Techniques for Anorectal Prolapse

Edited by

David Jayne
Department of Colorectal Surgery, Leeds General Hospital, Great George Street, Leeds, LS1 3EX, UK

Angelo Stuto
2nd Surgical Unit, "Ospedale S: maria degli Angeli", Pordenone, Italy

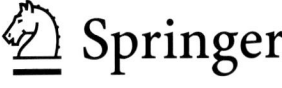

Springer

Editors
David Jayne
Department of Colorectal Surgery
Leeds General Hospital
Great George Street
Leeds, LS1 3EX
UK

Angelo Stuto
2nd Surgical Unit
"Ospedale S: Maria degli Angeli"
Pordenone
Italy

ISBN: 978-1-84800-904-2   e-ISBN: 978-1-84800-905-9
DOI: 10.1007/978-1-84800-905-9

British Library Cataloguing in Publication Data

Library of Congress Control Number: 2008941018

Printed on acid-free paper

Springer Science+Business Media
springer.com

Foreword

It has never been easy to introduce new concepts and therapeutic in-terventions into surgical practice. When attempting to do so, one is faced with the interagency of traditional dogma, which still in this era of evidence-based medicine tends to dominate the surgical thought process. This is particularly so in the area of coloproctology, where prejudice and personal opinion often influence objective analysis whenever tradition is challenged. A large body of literature on anorectal prolapse has accumulated over the years; although much is based on personal viewpoint rather than scientific evidence, it has nevertheless been passed down through the generations as ac-cepted wisdom and practice. As a consequence, it is a challenge to change the mindset of a generation of surgeons and to introduce new concepts and novel techniques which at first might appear to be a radical departure from conventional teaching.

It is obviously not possible to present the basis for the develop-ment of transanal stapling techniques for anorectal prolapse in this Foreword; this is dealt with in detail elsewhere in this book. The in-terested reader will have the opportunity to share in the new and emerging concepts surrounding anorectal prolapse and to deepen their understanding of the pathophysiology and basis for surgical correction. Although hemorrhoidal disease and external rectal prolapse have been known about for centuries, the understanding of internal rectal prolapse (intussusception) and rectocele has only really advanced with the emergence of radiological imaging tech-niques, such as defecography. With a heightened awareness of the condition, it has become apparent that the prevalence of sympto-matic anorectal prolapse is far more common than originally por-trayed, and that its impact on quality of life has been underestimated and undervalued. Perhaps for the first time, modern surgical tech-niques can now offer symptomatic improvement and enhanced qual-ity of life for those unfortunate enough to suffer with this chronic condition.

Historically, hemorrhoidal prolapse, internal and external rectal prolapse, and rectocele have been considered as separate clinical en-tities, with distinct etiologies. Modern think-ing and clinical observa-tion, however, would suggest that the different manifestations of anorectal prolapse in fact share a common pathophysiological basis. There is thus emerging a unified theory for anorectal prolapse.

Transanal Stapling for Anorectal Prolapse provides the reader with a clear overview of the pathophysiological basis of the disease and the evolution of transanal stapling tech-niques. Chapters have been contributed by an international panel of expert colorectal sur-geons to give a broad and comprehensive coverage of the subject. As well as covering the history and pathophysiology of anorectal prolapse, this book provides a structured approach to anorectal sta-pling techniques along with "tips and tricks" for success. This book will be an essential reference for all specialists with an interest in coloproctology.

Wien, Austria
Antonio Longo

v

Contents

Contributors

Steven Brown
Northern General Hospital, Sheffield, UK

Fabrice Corbisier
CH Notre-Dame et Reine, Fabiola, Belgium

Eloy Espin
Hospital Univeritari Vall, Barcelona, Spain

Franc Hetzer
Kantonsspital St. Gallen, St. Gallen, Switzerland

David Jayne
Academic Surgical Unit, St. James's University Hospital, Leeds, UK

V. Landolfi
General Surgery, "Landolfi"; Hospital, Solofra (AV), Italy

Leonardo Lenisa
Casa di Cura San Pio X, Milan, Italy

Antonio Longo
St. Elizabeth Hospital, Wien, Austria

Karen Nugent
Southampton General Hospital, Southampton, UK

Francois Pigot
Bagatelle-Maison de Sante, Talence Cedex, France

Roland Scherer
Krankenhaus Waldfriede, Berlin, Germany

Oliver Schwandner
Caritas Krankenhaus Str. Josef, Regensburg, Germany

Anthony Senagore
Department of Surgery, Medical University of Ohio, Toledo, OH, USA

Andrew Shorthouse
Northern General Hospital, Sheffield, UK

Angelo Stuto
2nd Surgical Unit, Ospedale S. Maria degli Angeli, Pordenone, Italy

Jean-Jacques Tuech
CHU Hopitaux de Rouen, Rouen, France

Introduction

David Jayne and Angelo Stuto

The first transanal stapling technique for the treatment of anorectal prolapse was presented at the 2nd World Congress of Coloproctology in Rome in 1998 by Dr. Antonio Longo [1]. This described a novel technique for the surgical correction of prolapsing hemorrhoids, originally referred to as procedure for prolapse and hemorrhoids (PPH) and more recently as stapled hemorrhoidopexy. Since that time, the technique has developed and gone on to enjoy tremendous success, due mainly to its benefits in reducing postoperative pain, shortening hospital stay, and achieving an earlier return to normal activities. Although a source of controversy in the early years, it has subsequently been subjected to critical appraisal and has provoked many randomized clinical trials, meta-analyses, and more recently in 2007 a favorable review from the National Institute for Health and Clinical Excellence (NICE) [2].

A natural evolution of stapled hemorrhoidopexy was its application to patients with obstructed defecation syndrome (ODS). This condition is common among multiparous women, and results from a dysfunctional pelvic floor giving rise to symptoms of constipation and an inability to satisfactorily evacuate the rectum. It is associated with characteristic anatomical abnormalities of the lower rectum, which impede the normal expulsion of feces. These abnormalities include rectocele formation, rectal intussusception (internal prolapse), and mucosal prolapse. The stapled transanal rectal resection (STARR) procedure is an extension of stapled hemorrhoidopexy, but instead of producing a mucosal resection of the hemorrhoidal prolapse it achieves a full-thickness resection of the lower rectum, incorporating any rectocele, intussusception, or prolapse. In this way, the anatomical obstruction to evacuation is removed, and normal defecatory function is restored. Although still a relatively new technique, the STARR procedure is attracting great interest among coloproctologists. This enthusiasm is fueled, at least in part, by encouraging early results which suggest a short-term efficacy of around 80% with acceptable rates of morbidity.

The time is now right for a book on transanal stapling techniques for anorectal prolapse. Both stapled hemorrhoidopexy and STARR have recently enjoyed widespread exposure and their application is spreading rapidly, particularly in Europe, but also across the rest of the world. However, many areas of controversy remain and warrant comprehensive discussion. Our current thinking on anorectal prolapse and its treatment has evolved significantly in recent years and this needs to be updated and documented.

The aims of this book are to fill a knowledge gap and to provide a comprehensive review of current thinking and practice in the management of anorectal prolapse, with emphasis on stapled hemorrhoidopexy for prolapsing hemorrhoids and the STARR procedure for ODS. This will be set against a historical background recording the development of the two procedures to put them in context and to provide further interest for the reader. In addition, it is hoped that the book will provide practical guidance in the application of

D. Jayne and A. Stuto (eds.), Transanal Stapling Techniques for Anorectal Prolapse,
DOI: 10.1007/978-1-84800-905-9_1, © Springer-Verlag London Limited 2009

the techniques with criteria for patient selection, tips, and tricks for obtaining the best outcomes, and how to avoid and deal with potential complications. Wherever possible, the views of the authors will be supported by evidence drawn from personal experience and the literature. The final section of the book will concentrate on unresolved controversies and suggest areas for further research and development.

It is hoped that this book will be of benefit to higher surgical trainees who are learning for the first time the complexities of proctological practice as well as established general surgeons and coloproctologists who encounter the conditions on a frequent basis. It is increasingly being recognized that anorectal prolapse is often one component of a more complex pelvic floor disorder, which necessitates multidisciplinary collaboration between coloproctologists, gynecologists, and urologists. This book may therefore also appeal to practitioners in these associated specialties.

The editors have been privileged to receive contributions from a dedicated and enthusiastic international panel of experts. It is hoped that the reader will benefit from their collective experience and insights into the rapidly evolving arena of transanal stapling for anorectal prolapse.

References

1. Longo A. Treatment of haemorrhoidal disease by reduction of mucosal and haemorrhoidal prolapse with a circular stapling device: a new procedure. Proceedings of the 6th World Congress of Endoscopic Surgery. Rome, Italy, 1998, June 3–6, pp 777–84
2. National Institute for Health and Clinical Excellence (2007) Stapled haemorrhoidopexy for the treatment of haemorrhoids: NICE technology appraisal guidance 128. Available at http://www.nice.org.uk/TA128

Chapter 1
Historical Background: Treatments for Hemorrhoids and ODS Prior to Transanal Stapling Techniques

Longo, L. Lenisa, and V. Landolfi

Abstract Over the past decade several innovations in surgical technology have tried to address the painful anodermal wounds and protracted recovery associated with conventional excisional hemorrhoidectomy. Of these, only the stapled hemorrhoidopexy has achieved recognition as a viable alternative. However, the introduction of stapled hemorrhoidopexy into routine clinical practice was not without controversy. In this chapter, we describe the rationale underlying the technique and discuss the historical background to its eventual acceptance. In addition, we present the evolution of a novel technique, stapled transanal rectal resection (STARR) for the treatment of obstructed defecation syndrome (ODS). This was inspired by the success of stapled hemorrhoidopexy together with the observation that symptoms of rectal outlet obstruction could be improved by resection of the redundant distal rectum. The concept of internal rectal prolapse as the primary etiology underlying ODS is presented.

Treatment of Hemorrhoids Prior to PPH

Hemorrhoidal tissue is a normal component of the anal canal and consists of a vascular plexus supported by smooth muscle and connective tissue. If the vascular plexus becomes engorged or prolapses it can cause symptoms of bleeding, pruritis, pain, and disordered evacuation. Under normal conditions, it provides a compressible lining that assists in closure of the anus and the maintenance of continence.

The prevalence of hemorrhoidal symptoms is high in all populations [1, 2]. Estimates of prevalence in the UK population range from 4.4 to 36.4% [3] with approximately 23,000 hemorrhoidal procedures performed per annum [4]. Reports from US and UK physicians indicate 1,177 and 1,123 per 100,000 consults per year, respectively, with hemorrhoidal complaints [5]. Both genders suffer from the disease, but there is a slightly higher tendency in males for recurrent symptoms [6], with 10–20% of patients with recurrent symptoms requiring surgery [7].

Internal hemorrhoids are usually classified on the basis of the extent of associated prolapse. First-degree hemorrhoids bleed because of vascular congestion and mucosal trauma on defecation, but are not prolapsed. Second-degree hemorrhoids prolapse under straining but reduce spontaneously. In third-degree hemorrhoids, manual reduction of the prolapse is required, while in fourth-degree hemorrhoids there is a dislocation of the vascular pedicles out of the anal canal.

The initial treatment for first- and second-degree hemorrhoids includes alterations in lifestyle, diet and bowel habits, stool softeners, and topical ointments. Persistent symptoms may be treated by a variety of techniques, which share a common aim: to produce a controlled and localized destruction of the hemorrhoidal tissue resulting in fibrosis and fixation of the hemorrhoidal plexuses. Rubber band ligation involves the application of rubber bands to the mucosa of the upper anorectum, above the dentate line, using either grasping forceps or

D. Jayne and A. Stuto (eds.), *Transanal Stapling Techniques for Anorectal Prolapse,*
DOI: 10.1007/978-1-84800-905-9_1, © Springer-Verlag London Limited 2009

suction applicator. Injection sclerotherapy consists of an injection of a sclerosant, usually phenol in almond oil, into the submucosa of the upper anal canal. Infrared coagulation utilizes the fibrotic effects of small burns, while cryotherapy causes mucosal necrosis by freezing and can be used alone or in combination with rubber band ligation. Although all these procedures may be performed in the outpatient clinic their durability, particularly in grade ≥2 prolapse, is questionable. Many patients require multiple sessions and there is a high recurrence rate. Although widely thought of as safe procedures, serious side effects have been reported. Nonetheless, rubber band ligation and sclerotherapy remain popular because of their ease of application and their acceptability by patients. These treatments will continue to play an important part in the treatment of early-grade prolapse for the foreseeable future, regardless of new surgical interventions.

Traditional excisional surgery for hemorrhoids aimed at debulking the hemorrhoidal mass using a variety of dissection techniques and means of hemostasis. In this regard, the term hemorrhoidectomy is appropriately applied. However, any excisional surgery which involves the lower anal canal will inevitably leave a painful anodermal wound as the lining of the anal canal below the dentate line is exquisitively sensitive, which contrasts to the relatively insensate mucosa of the upper anorectum. The resulting painful anal wound has been the main limitation of most previous hemorrhoidectomy techniques and the main driving force for developments in surgical approach.

Circumferential closed hemorrhoidectomy was proposed by Whitehead in 1887 [8] and involved excision of the hemorrhoidal pedicles followed by closure of the wound by suturing the rectal mucosa to the residual anodermal tissue. Although it dealt adequately with large prolapsing hemorrhoids, it was limited by the complexity of the procedure, the high postoperative pain, and frequent anodermal complications including stricture formation and ectropion.

In 1947 Milligan–Morgan [9] described an open excisional hemorrhoidectomy, which has remained the most popular procedure for hemorrhoids in Europe until recent years. In the original description, the hemorrhoids were exposed with clamps to reveal the so-called Milligan–Morgan triangle.

The prolapsing piles were excised up to the inner anal canal with ligation of the pedicles to minimize bleeding. In an attempt to reduce postoperative sepsis the surgical wound was left "open" to heal by secondary intention. This occurred over a period of 3–4 weeks, during which the patient was left with a painful, open wound.

In an attempt to overcome the troublesome postoperative pain, in 1956 Parks [10] proposed a submucosal hemorrhoidal excision with high ligation of the pedicles and subsequent reconstruction of the mucosal and submucosal layers. A similar technique of closed hemorrhoidectomy was subsequently described in 1959 by Fergusson [11] and to date remains the preferred procedure in Northern America.

With advances in surgical technology, and in particular the development of new modalities for hemostasis came the opportunity to improve on previous excisional hemorrhoidectomy techniques. Thus, hemorrhoidectomy has been performed with diathermy coagulation [12], laser [13], harmonic scalpel [14, 15], and radiofrequency coagulation [16, 17]. Harmonic scalpel and radiofrequency ablation take advantage of the improved hemostasis and reduced tissue trauma, and have been proposed as useful techniques to facilitate day-case hemorrhoidectomy. Although they improve operative hemostasis and probably reduce the incidence of postoperative bleeding, their effect on postoperative pain reduction is controversial [18–23]. Similarly, although supporters of laser ablation and diathermy dissection claim a reduction in postoperative pain, the evidence is unconvincing with other randomized trials failing to show a clear difference compared to traditional hemorrhoidectomy [24–26].

In 1995 Morinaga proposed a novel approach to hemorrhoidal treatment; hemorrhoidal artery ligation under Doppler guidance [27]. A fenestrated anoscope and Doppler ultrasound were used to place three to six transfixion sutures around branches of the superior hemorrhoidal artery. This was a nonresectional technique, proposed for the treatment of third- and fourth-degree piles, which relied purely on a vascular etiology of hemorrhoids. Initial results appeared positive, and the technique had the advantage of being applied in the outpatient setting. However, skepticism exists as to the long-term efficacy of the procedure, for which there is a lack of evidence from randomized trials.

There is also the concern that the procedure does not address the anodermal prolapse component of hemorrhoidal disease, although there have been attempts to address this in various modifications of the original technique.

Treatment of ODS Prior to STARR

Stapled Transanal Rectal Resection (STARR) is a relatively new and novel surgical treatment for obstructed defecation syndrome (ODS). It indications include ODS symptoms in the presence of internal rectal prolapse/intussusception with or without an associated rectocele. It aims to produce a surgical correction of these anatomical entities using a transanal resectional technique. In this regard it is a unique surgical approach for which there is not a good historical comparator. Moreover, some authorities take the view that obstructed defecation should be managed by nonoperative means, which makes STARR a controversial treatment modality within the spectrum of pelvic floor disorders. For these reasons, a historical overview is presented of different modalities previously or currently used in the treatment of ODS.

NonSurgical Treatment of ODS

The first-line treatment for constipated patients should address dietary habits leading to slow colonic transit. Patients should be advised about the importance of adequate fluid intake (2–3 l daily) and the benefits of a high-fiber diet in relation to increased colonic transit time. Osmotic stool softeners may be helpful and can be used fairly freely with intermittent use of stimulant laxatives as necessary. The prolonged use of stimulant laxatives is to be discouraged if at all possible.

Pelvic floor rehabilitation has a role in rectal evacuatory disorders, such as anismus and pelvic dyssynergia, as a modality for sensory and motor retraining. Various techniques have been described for this purpose including biofeedback therapy, electrostimulation, and pelviperineal physiokinesis. Biofeedback therapy aims to re-establish conscious control of physiological mechanisms that have been lost as a consequence of rectal prolapse, neuropathy, trauma, or other systemic disease. In last decades, biofeedback has been widely tested for

the treatment of urinary and fecal incontinence, but only relatively recently has its role been explored in the treatment of constipation and rectal evacuation [28]. Pelvic floor retraining is undertaken with the use of an endoanal probe that transduce signals from electromyography or anorectal manometry to an external device as a visual scale, giving the trainee information about ongoing pelvic activity during exercises to improve conscious appreciation. Biofeedback provides useful information regarding agonistic and antagonistic physiological responses, facilitates improved control of sphincter relaxation/contraction, enhances appropriate muscle recruitment, and improves rectal compliance and sensibility. Advocates of biofeedback claim an improvement in rectal perception, voluntary motor control, colonic motility, and normalization of the rectoanal inhibitory reflex [29, 30]. Treatment schedules vary widely with sessions ranging from 15 to 90 min, two or three times per week, over several months. Compliance to treatment and recurrence of symptoms on long-term follow-up are the main drawbacks of the technique.

Electrical stimulation techniques are based on their ability to facilitate voluntary motor activity and improve neuromuscular control. These procedures aim to improve the patient's perception of defecatory function and to augment muscular tone and strength. As a consequence, it is claimed that they achieve an improvement of rectoanal coordination, normalization of rectal sensitivity, and resetting of neurosacral reflexes [31]. Pelviperineal physiokinesis may be used in combination with biofeedback and electrical stimulation to improve the effects of rehabilitation and to prevent recurrences at the end of treatment.

Surgical Treatment of Rectocele

Historically, rectoceles have been considered as herniations of the anterior rectal wall into posterior vaginal space and have been treated both by gynecologists and coloproctologists using either a transvaginal, transperineal, or transanal approach. Regardless of the surgical approach, the aim has been to reduce the rectal herniation rather than correct any associated rectal evacuatory dysfunction. Indications for surgery have included perineal discomfort and symptoms related to vaginal "bulging," dysperunia, and associated genital prolapse with urinary and defecatory dysfunction. To date, the majority of women with symptomatic rectoceles present to the gynecologist or urogynecologist in the first instance, with the preferred treatment more a matter of personal preference than based on clinical evidence. It should be noted that the finding of a small rectocele is not uncommon in the normal female population and is not in itself an indication for surgical intervention.

The transvaginal approach is performed by incision of the posterior vaginal wall to expose the rectovaginal space which is dissected to allow reduction of the herniated portion of rectum. The rectovaginal space and the perineal body are reconstructed, traditionally by suture placation, and the posterior vaginal wall repaired. Additional procedures may be performed to reduce the risk of rectocele recurrence, and include levatorplasty, interposition of a mesh (resorbable, permanent, biologic, etc.), and resuspension of vaginal stump. Associated genital prolapse or cystocele can be treated at the same time either transvaginally or with a combined open or laparoscopic abdominal procedure.

The transperineal approach is similar, but access to the rectovaginal space is obtained through a transverse perineal incision with dissection of perineal body. Again the rectocele is reduced posteriorly and the rectovaginal space reconstructed using similar techniques.

The disadvantage of both transvaginal and transperineal approaches lies in the persistent redundancy of the lower rectum and the accompanying fibrosis of rectovaginal space, which may exacerbate symptoms of rectal outlet obstruction.

The transanal approach tends to be preferred by general surgeons and coloproctologists. A variety of procedures and subsequent modifications have been proposed for rectocele repair. Block [32] described direct suture of the anterior wall with full-thickness stitches placed 1 cm apart to cover the entire defect. Although he reported a 100% patient satisfaction, some 77% of patients were left with a residual rectocele albeit asymptomatic. Sullivan described an original technique for transanal rectocele repair, which was subsequently modified by Sarles and Khubchandani [33, 34]. This involved a transverse incision above the dentate line with creation of an anterior mucosal-submucosal rectal flap upward to the apex of rectocele. Plication of

the rectal wall defect was performed and the redundant mucosa excised. Generally, the technique resulted in a reasonable improvement in defecatory function in the short term, but with deteriorating efficacy with time such that only 50% of patients remained asymptomatic at 5-year follow-up. The technique did nothing to amend any posterior rectal wall prolapse that might accompany the rectocele, and this may explain to some extent the poor long-term outcomes.

Surgical Treatment for Rectal Prolapse/ Intussusception

Internal rectal prolapse and intussusception are recognized causes of outlet obstruction. Their true prevalence is thought to be underestimated as the majority of patients do not seek medical attention. Historically, the surgical approach to their repair has been either by transanal, transperineal, or transabdominal operations, a full description of which is outside the scope of this chapter.

Similarly, a wide variety of procedures have been proposed for the treatment of full-thickness external rectal prolapse. As yet, there is no consensus as to the best treatment for external prolapse, although the results of randomized controlled trials (the PROSPER study) are eagerly awaited. Probably the best known perineal procedure is that first proposed by Delorme, who described a transanal resection of the rectal mucosa with subsequent plication of muscular rectal wall and sutured anastomosis of residual rectal mucosa to anal mucosa. It is a safe and easy procedure, and its low morbidity makes it an attractive option in the medically unfit patient. However, it is associated with a high recurrence rate of 30–40% on long-term follow-up. An intrarectal variation of the Delorme procedure, the so-called internal Delorme's, has been proposed as a treatment for internal rectal prolapse and intussusception. However, restricted access to the anal canal makes this a difficult and frequently bloody procedure. Altemeier proposed a transperineal proctosigmoidectomy with coloanal anastomosis for the treatment of external rectal prolapse, the anastomosis being performed either by suture or more recently by a stapling technique. Transabdominal operations for external prolapse may be undertaken using either an open or laparoscopic technique and include suture rectopexy (Moschovitz, Orr-Loygue with fascial tapes, Ripstein with sacral fixation), mesh rectopexy (Wells-Ellis, Nicholls), and resection-rectopexy (Frykman-Golberg et al.). However, these techniques have limited efficacy when only internal prolapse/intussusception is present. New procedures specifically aimed at the treatment of internal prolapse associated with obstructed defecation include laparoscopic ventral rectopexy [35, 36] and the EXPRESS Procedure [37]. The efficacy of these techniques on long-term follow-up remains to be seen.

The Development of Transanal Stapling Techniques

Our knowledge of hemorrhoidal disease has evolved over the years in line with a better understanding of the normal and pathological anatomical and physiological states. Three abnormalities are commonly encountered in patients with symptomatic hemorrhoids: abnormal prolapse of anorectal mucosa; distal displacement and venous engorgement of the hemorrhoidal plexus; and the presence of external skin tags.

The vascular theory attributes hemorrhoidal disease to pathological varicose dilatation of the anal canal vascular plexuses. This theory is largely viewed as being oversimplified and is longer considered as a credible explanation [38, 39]. This view is supported by epidemiological studies which have failed to show a correlation between venous outflow in portal hypertension and hemorrhoidal engorgement [40, 41]. Anorectal varices linked to portal hypertension and primary hemorrhoidal disease are now classified as separate entities [42, 43].

Previous theories linking hemorrhoidal symptoms to hypertrophy and hyperplasia of the anal cushions have been disproved by studies which have failed to show any histological difference in anal canal tissue obtained from patients with hemorrhoids and healthy subjects [44].

In 1975, Thomson described the anatomy of the anal cushions and defined their role in the mechanism of continence [38]. His observations are fundamental to our current understanding of the pathogenesis of hemorrhoidal disease. The anal cushions, commonly distributed in three segments around the anal canal, are part of the normal anatomy. They are formed by arteriolar and venular microscopic anastomosis within the anal canal, supported by smooth muscle and connective tissue [45]. The anal mucosa and the anal cushions receive their blood supply from the superior, middle, and inferior rectal arteries. The blood flow provided by these arteries is excessive for normal nutritional needs, but serves the additional purpose of allowing rapid engorgement of the cushions as required. This augments the function of the internal cushions in maintaining anal continence [44]. Excessive ablation of the hemorrhoidal cushions, as may result from hemorrhoidectomy, will thus have a negative impact on normal continence to gas and liquid stools [46].

Thomson's hypothesis suggests that it is the prolapse of the anal cushions and rectal mucosa which is the main determinant of symptom hemorrhoids. This concept also underlies the theoretical basis for stapled hemorrhoidopexy. It is believed that chronic straining to defecate results in fragmentation of the anal supporting tissues, the so-called Trietz's ligaments, with accompanying prolapse of the anorectal mucosa and hemorrhoids. Moreover, if Park's ligaments are torn, there will be a distal sliding of the anoderm as well. Prolapse of the anal cushions causes an alteration in their vascular anatomy, with stretching of the superior rectal arterioles and kinking of the vascular connections between the internal and external vascular plexuses of the middle and inferior vessels. This altered anatomy may be exaggerated by an associated increase in sphincter tone. These vascular modifications impair normal venous drainage, resulting in dilatation of the anal cushions, edema, and hypoxia. The hypoxic acidosis and the accompanying inflammation then activate coagulative mechanisms leading to hemorrhoidal thrombosis. The pathogenesis of hemorrhoidal disease is thus believed to be linked to a condition of venous stasis rather than a primary disease of the hemorrhoidal tissue per se, even though no correlation has been established between hemorrhoidal disease and venous disorders, such as varices and varicocele [40, 47]. While prolapse of the anal mucosa is very common among subjects over 50 years of age [48], it only becomes symptomatic in a low percentage of cases [49]. This might appear to support the idea that mucosal prolapse and hemorrhoids are not closely linked. However, hemorrhoids rarely develop in the absence of pro-lapse, and it is likely that the prolapse is the initiating event which only becomes symptomatic when complications supervene.

Although the majority of patients complain of vascular complications related to hemorrhoidal prolapse, other symptoms may also be present. Minor incontinence or soiling may be a feature attributable to anorectal prolapse, giving rise to pruritis ani. This is exacerbated by displacement of the sensitive anorectal mucosa which is important for the normal rectoanal inhibitory reflex and anal sampling [46].

superior rectal artery in addition to resuspending and fixing the prolapsed tissue to the underlying anorectal muscle. This approach restores the normal anatomical relationship between the anal mucosa and the anal sphincter, leading to an improvement in venous return. It is also reasonable to assume that interruption of the terminal branches of the superior rectal artery, by reducing blood flow to the submucosal spaces of the anal canal, helps in controlling hemorrhoidal bleeding [45, 49]. The excision of redundant mucohemorrhoidal tissue may also be beneficial to outlet transit of the fecal

The Concept of Mucosal Prolapsectomy and Hemorrhoidopexy

Assuming that mucosal prolapse is the etiology underlying hemorrhoidal disease, then attempts to cure the condition must be directed at correction or removal of the prolapse itself rather than excision of the hemorrhoids. In pursue of this goal, a technique has been developed, stapled hemorrhoidopexy, which corrects mucosal and hemorrhoidal prolapse by means of excision of a transverse band of distal rectal mucosa at the level of the anorectal junction. Excision of the mucosa at this level interrupts the terminal branches of the

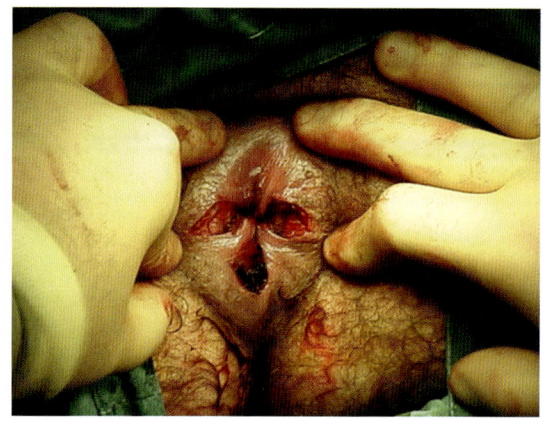

Fig. 1.1. The "clover-leaf" appearance of the anus with painful open anodermal wounds following conventional open hemorrhoidectomy

A   B

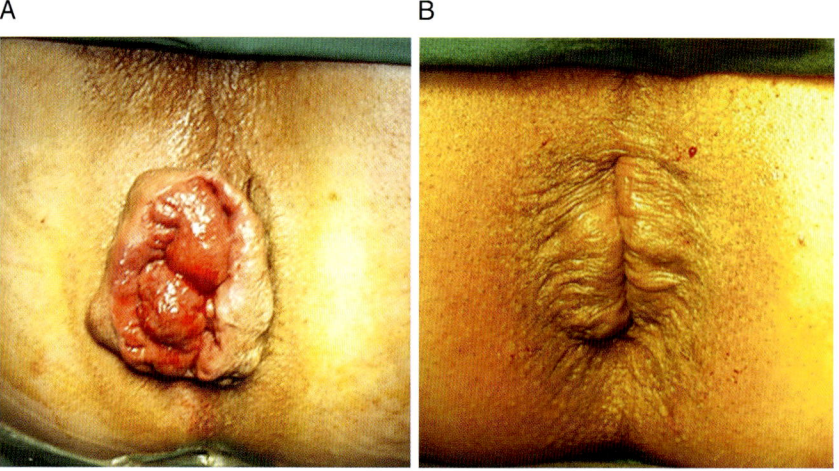

Fig. 1.2. (**a**) Fourth-degree hemorrhoidal prolapse; (**b**) the end result following stapled hemorrhoidopexy, with no anodermal wounds. The prolapsing piles have been reduced and the stapled anastomosis is above the level of the sensitive dentate line

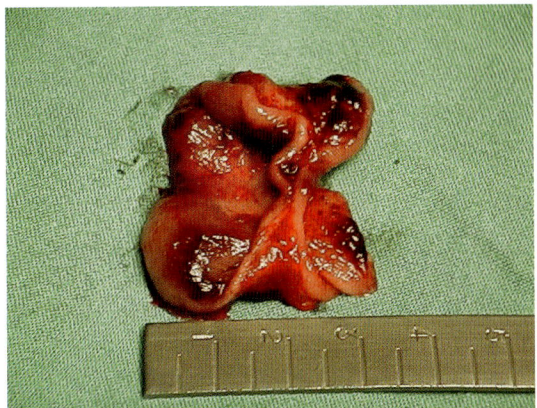

FIG. 1.3. A complete submucosal resection doughnut of the distal rectum and hemorrhoids following stapled hemorrhoidopexy

mass, reducing friction and trauma to the anal canal lining during the process of defecation. Restoration of normal anorectal anatomy also helps to preserve the sensory functions of the anal mucosa which are integral to normal defecation and continence [50].

The end result of mucosal prolapsectomy is an end-to-end mucomucosal anastomosis at the anorectal junction, which is relatively devoid of somatic pain fibers. This contrasts to the open anodermal wounds associated with conventional excisional hemorrhoidectomy (Figs. 1.1–1.3).

It should be stressed that the procedure being proposed is no longer a hemorrhoidectomy. The technique resuspends the mucosal prolapse but leaves the hemorrhoidal cushions intact. It is in effect a rectal mucosal prolapsectomy and combined hemorrhoidopexy. Residual external skin tags may be removed at the end of procedure if cosmesis is an issue, but the hemorrhoidal cushions of the inner anal canal must be preserved.

The full description of the PPH stapled hemorrhoidopexy technique is provided in Chap. 6.

Stapled Hemorrhoidopexy (PPH): The Early Years and Controversy

The introduction of the PPH technique was followed by initial positive reports from a number of centers in Italy and Europe [51–54]. These studies suggested that the technique was feasible and safe, and that postoperative complications were comparable to conventional excisional hemorrhoidectomy. In addition, there was the added advantage of reduced postoperative pain and earlier return to normal activities.

In 2000 two randomized trials comparing stapled hemorrhoidopexy to excision hemorrhoidectomy were published in *The Lancet*. One was conducted by Rowsell and colleagues [55] and concluded that stapled hemorrhoidopexy resulted in shorter inpatient stay, less postoperative pain, and quicker return to work. Symptoms of prolapse, discharge, and bleeding were controlled in all patients at 6 weeks' follow-up. The second was conducted by Mehigan and coworkers [56] and similarly concluded that the stapling technique was associated with shorter anesthetic time, less postoperative pain, and quicker return to normal function. Early and late complications and functional outcomes were comparable to excision hemorrhoidectomy.

However, the initial enthusiasm for stapled hemorrhoidopexy was halted some months later by a publication in the same journal from Cheetham and colleagues at St Mark's Hospital, London [57]. This reported the results of a randomized trial comparing stapled hemorrhoidopexy with conventional hemorrhoidectomy, which was terminated early due to unacceptable levels of postoperative pain and fecal urgency in five patients following stapled hemorrhoidopexy. As a consequence of this publication, concern was expressed among the colorectal fraternity, with opinion divided regarding the safety of the new stapling procedure.

Attempts to analyze the reasons for the pain and urgency reported in the Cheetham paper have failed to come up with a simple explanation. The patients were all operated on by a single surgeon, and this may have had some effect. The study protocol included the excision of external skin tags which may have explained some of the postoperative pain, but would not have explained the reported late pain and urgency. In two of the patients the staple line was recorded at 1 cm above the dentate line, which may be considered too low, especially when the patients were males who normally have a longer anal canal. Histological examination of the resection specimens revealed the presence of smooth muscle fibers, but this is a common finding following both stapled hemorrhoidopexy and conventional hemorrhoidectomy [58] and results from inclusion of smooth muscle fibers of the lower rectum which has no impact on functional outcome [59]. The stretching effect of the 35-mm anal dilator included in the PPH01™ kit on the anal sphincters has been postulated by some as a potential cause of muscle fragmentation, but this hypothesis has been largely discounted by subsequent studies demonstrating no effect on sphincter morphology. The most likely variable responsible for poor outcome seems to be the operating surgeon [58] which underlines the importance of adequate training prior to taking on the procedure.

The impact of the adverse reporting from the St. Marks' group was heightened by case reports of serious complications from other institutions. These included the report by Molloy and Kingsmore [60] of life-threatening pelvic sepsis after stapled hemorrhoidopexy in a young male, despite the procedure having been uneventful and the staple line found to be intact. A further episode of retroperitoneal sepsis after stapled hemorrhoidopexy was reported from Singapore [61], which was successfully managed by conservative means. Three rectal perforations requiring colostomy, one complete rectal obstruction, one large retro-rectal hematoma, and one lethal sepsis due to Fournier's gangrene were reported by Herold from a German survey of 4,635 stapled hemorrhoidopexies [62]. Rectal perforation was reported from Taiwan [63], and rectal perforation, retropneumoperitoneum, and pneumomediastinum from Italy [64] in a case where an imperfect, modified PPH technique resulted in a disastrous complication.

These isolated cases, when taken together, not unreasonably attracted criticism and skepticism from a general surgical and colorectal community unfamiliar with PPH and resulted in a period of reflection.

The Acceptance of Stapled Hemorrhoidopexy (PPH)

The period of reflection and caution for PPH as a consequence of adverse reporting was transient and subsequently overwhelmed by positive experiences from many centers worldwide. In 2001 the St Mark's group published the definitive results of the randomized trial on PPH vs. excision hemorrhoidectomy [65], which somehow counterbalanced the negative results of its previous publication [57]. This was the first report demonstrating that stapled hemorrhoidopexy could be performed as a day-case procedure: stapled hemorrhoidopexy was favorable in terms of reduced pain (despite concurrent excision of skin tags), quicker return to work (10 vs.14 days), and similar patient satisfaction scores. However, the authors concluded that long-term symptomatic relief was poor when compared with conventional hemorrhoidectomy, particularly in patients with external hemorrhoids. This view was not shared by other surgeons experienced in PPH who were of the opinion that "initial concerns that staplers are applicable only for early haemorrhoids and not third- or fourth- degree haemorrhoids appear to be unfounded" [66]. Gradually, as experience with the stapling technique increased, colorectal surgeons became more confident with the procedure. In 2003 Lehur [67] declared that PPH was a satisfying procedure for both the surgeon and the patient as hemorrhoids are treated fast and effectively, with minimum postoperative pain, little nursing, and faster return to normal activities through a restoration of normal anatomy and with sparing of the hemorrhoidal cushions.

Between 2001 and 2006 a large body of evidence, largely in support of stapled hemorrhoidopexy, accumulated from case series, consensus papers, systemic reviews, and randomized controlled trials. A thorough review of the literature on stapled hemorrhoidopexy (PPH) is provided in Chap. 8. A recent publication by Tjandra et al. [68] involved a meta-analysis of 25 randomized, controlled trials performed up until 2007. This careful analysis of the evidence concluded that stapled hemorrhoidopexy was superior to conventional hemorrhoidectomy in terms of shorter operative time, reduced hospital stay, less postoperative pain and analgesic requirement, faster recovery and return to work, quicker wound healing, and increased patient satisfaction.

To date over 7 million PPH procedures have been performed worldwide and in Italy, where the procedure was invented, stapled hemorrhoidopexy now accounts for over 60% of all hemorrhoidal interventions.

In 2007 the National Institute for Health and Clinical Excellence (NICE) in the U.K. produced an updated technology appraisal for PPH [4] stating that "Stapled haemorrhoidopexy, using a circular stapler specifically developed for haemorrhoidopexy, is recommended as an option for people in whom surgical intervention is considered appropriate for the treatment of prolapsed internal haemorrhoids". It confirmed previous positive findings of reduced postoperative pain and earlier return to normal activities. No difference was found in the rate or nature of postoperative complications, with a trend for less bleeding following stapled hemorrhoidopexy and fewer wound-related problems. A cost-effectiveness analysis considering short-term usage of health resources concluded that there was little difference between stapled hemorrhoidopexy and conventional hemorrhoidectomy, with the cost of the stapling device being offset by the reduced length of hospital stay. The only caveat relating to stapled hemorrhoidopexy was an increased incidence of recurrent prolapse on long-term follow-up. This was mirrored by an increased rate of reinterventions following stapled hemorrhoidopexy, although this did not pose any greater risk than reinterventions after conventional hemorrhoidectomy. The guidance concluded that stapled hemorrhoidopexy was "an appropriate use of NHS resources."

The Recognition of Abnormalities Associated with ODS

Constipation can be considered a social disease due to its prevalence in an otherwise healthy population. It is responsible for a variety of symptoms which have a negative impact on an individual's quality of life.

Obstructed defecation syndrome (ODS) refers to an inability to achieve satisfactory defecation as consequence of rectal outlet disturbance. Pelvic dyssynergia or anismus has previously been considered to be a leading cause of ODS. Other conditions such as rectocele, rectal intussusception, enterocele, descending perineum, and genital prolapse were regarded as secondary anatomical entities which coexisted in patients with ODS. This concept is supported to some degree by findings of similar anatomical defects in otherwise healthy patients without ODS. Moreover, the complexity of pelvic floor disorders is poorly understood, and further confusion arises due to differing opinions from coloproctologists and urogynecologists.

A unitary vision is often lacking, but is needed for the correct interpretation and classification of pelvic floor dysfunction.

In an attempt to address this issue one of the authors (A.L.) undertook a series of anatomical, radiological, and clinical studies. The results may help our understanding of the mechanisms underlying ODS and act as a guide for surgical treatment; the findings are summarized later.

Cadaver Dissections

Twenty-five cadaveric dissections were performed in 3 males and 22 females, ranging from 19 to 94 years of age. All rectal and uro-gynecological conditions were recorded. Four had undergone previous hysterectomy (with vaginal vault prolapse in 2); four had anterior and posterior colpocele and uterine prolapse; ten had a rectocele, rectal intussusceptions, or external rectal prolapse; seven were otherwise free of pelvic disease. Fresh dissection was performed in a mixed group of ten cadavers, while frozen cadaveric dissection was performed in the remaining 15 (in nine cases a balloon inflated with 400 ml of water had previously been inserted in the rectum).

In fresh dissection where a rectocele, rectal intussusceptions, or external rectal prolapse was present, the rectal portion lying beneath the sacropubic line was larger than controls, with a mean value of 4.2 cm (range: 2.4–7.3 cm), and the distal rectum was hypermobile. No difference in this length was detected between cases with rectocele, intussusceptions, or rectal prolapse: all cases showed a prolapse of the distal rectum to varying degrees. In cases where a rectocele was present, a thinning of the rectal wall was noted (to less than 25% of the normal rectal wall thickness), and in three cases this also involved the vaginal layer. After posterior dissection of the vaginal layer a balloon was introduced in the rectum and filled with 400 ml of water: in cases with rectocele a dilatation of the rectal ampulla was observed, while in controls the balloon filled the rectum in a longitudinal manner. This observation was confirmed ex vivo on explanted rectums.

Fresh and frozen dissections of cadavers with genital or vaginal vault prolapse showed that a concomitant rectal prolapse was to a certain extent always present, either involving the whole rectum

Fig. 1.4. Cadaveric dissection reveals thinning of the muscular layer of the anterior rectum and rectovaginal septum. *r* rectum, *v* vagina, *b* bladder

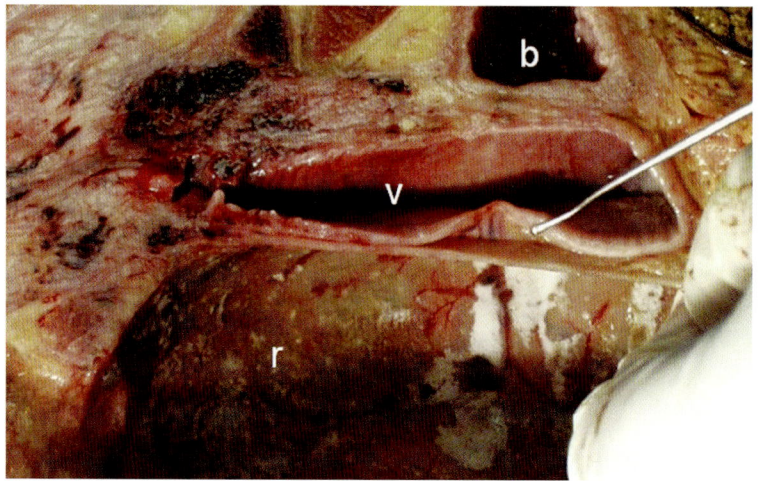

or isolated to the anterior rectal wall. In these cases, proximal traction on the vaginal vault resulted in a resuspension of the rectal prolapse.

Microscopic evaluation of rectocele specimens revealed that the rectal muscular layer was thinned and partially replaced by fibrous tissue. This alteration in rectal wall morphology was found mainly in the longitudinal layer of the anterolateral wall and was only detected circumferentially around the rectum in a minority of cases (Fig. 1.4).

It was concluded from these studies that:

- rectum in a minority of cases Rectocele and rectal intussusception are characterized by a stretching of distal rectum which appears to result in distal rectal prolapse.
- Rectoceles differ only in the accompanying alteration of the muscular layer of the rectal wall.
- Uterovaginal prolapse is associated with a concomitant descent of the rectum, particularly that of the anterior rectal wall.

Imaging in Patients with ODS

Ultrasonography

The authors have undertaken transrectal ultrasound examination in a series of patients with clinically detectable rectocele. Characteristically, there is a thinning or relative absence of the muscular layer of the rectum starting approximately 1 cm above the proximal extent of the internal sphincter muscle. This is most readily appreciated anterolaterally, but may also extend to some degree circumferentially.

Radiology

X-rays of the empty rectum which had been outlined with barium were taken of 220 patients with ODS and clinical evidence of rectocele, rectal intussusceptions, or external rectal prolapse and compared with control x-rays taken from patients undergoing imaging for other colonic disease. Patients with rectocele and/or intussusception had a larger amount of rectum beneath the sacropubic line. It was notable that rectocele and intussusception could not be distinguished from each other when the rectum was empty. The impression was that of a "floppy rectum" with distal rectum prolapse. An increased "mobility" of the rectal wall could readily be appreciated at fluoroscopy by the insertion of an examining finger.

To further evaluate the functional consequences of rectoceles and rectal intussusception patients were analyzed by modified defecography. Contrast medium was inserted into the bladder and vagina, and the sigmoid colon was filled via a rectal catheter leaving the rectum empty. Sequential x-rays were taken every 10 s and cinedefecography performed once the urge to defecate was experienced. Barium was found to either flow freely from the sigmoid colon to the anus, or was impeded at certain levels as it passed through the rectum corresponding to points of intussusception, which were present even at rest. In the filled rectum, the intussusception or internal prolapse disappeared upon straining to defecate by one of three mechanisms, either acting in isolation or together:

• Transverse distension with the formation of a rectocele
• Longitudinal stretching of the rectum manifest as perineal descent
• Expulsion of the prolapse through the anus forming an external rectal prolapse

The first mechanism was restricted to females, with the depth of the resultant rectocele being related to the thinning of the muscular layer of the rectal wall present on ultrasound. The second mechanism occurred independent of sex and did not appear to be associated with the length of rectum lying beneath the sacropubic line. The third mechanism was found more frequently in males.

Other frequent radiological findings observed during defecatory straining included reorientation of the vagina to approximate a horizontal position, deepening of the Pouch of Douglas often with associated enterocele or sigmoidocele, and perineal descent greater that 5 cm. These findings were associated with postdefecatory residual barium retention of 20% or higher.

The authors believe that damage to the muscular layer of the distal rectum results in an inability of the rectum to maintain intraluminal pressure during defecation. In this situation, extraluminal pressure is required to achieve defecation, which is derived through horizontal and posterior displacement of the vagina and accompanying descent of the Pouch of Douglas. This altered state of pelvic anatomy may either reduce spontaneously on cessation of straining, or if chronic may become stabilized over time. In this setting, hyperdescent of the perineum may also act as a partial compensatory mechanism, allowing longitudinal distension of the distal rectal prolapse and facilitating rectal evacuation.

Based on these observations, it is believed that the symptoms of obstructed defecation syndrome can be explained on the basis of a redundancy of the distal rectum, which functionally may act in one or more of the following ways:

• Rectoanal intussusception impedes the normal flow of fecal material toward the anus and prevents the initiation of defecation
• Internal rectal prolapse or circumferential rectoanal intussusception interrupts rectal evacuation
• The anterior rectal wall bulges into the vagina forming a rectocele and in so doing the rectum comes to lie transversely across the pelvic floor
• Feces becomes entrapped into the rectocele by early rectoanal intussusception

Figures 1.5 and 1.6 demonstrate the characteristic anatomical abnormalities demonstrated on dynamic defecography and MRI in patients with ODS. Figures 1.7 and 1.8 show the intraoperative appearances of a rectocele and anorectal prolapse.

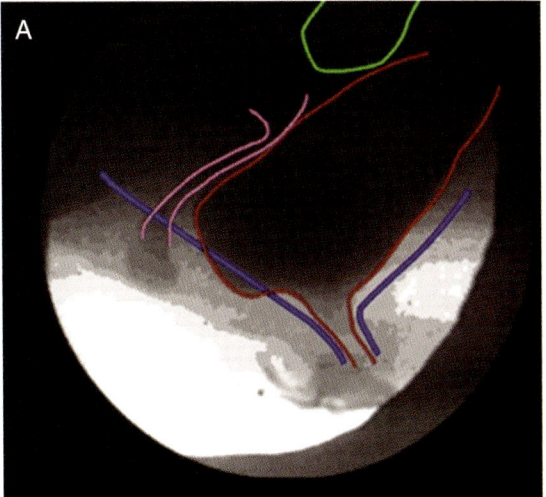
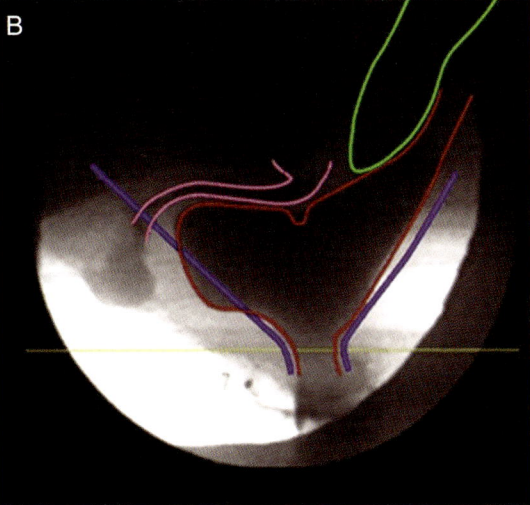

(continued)

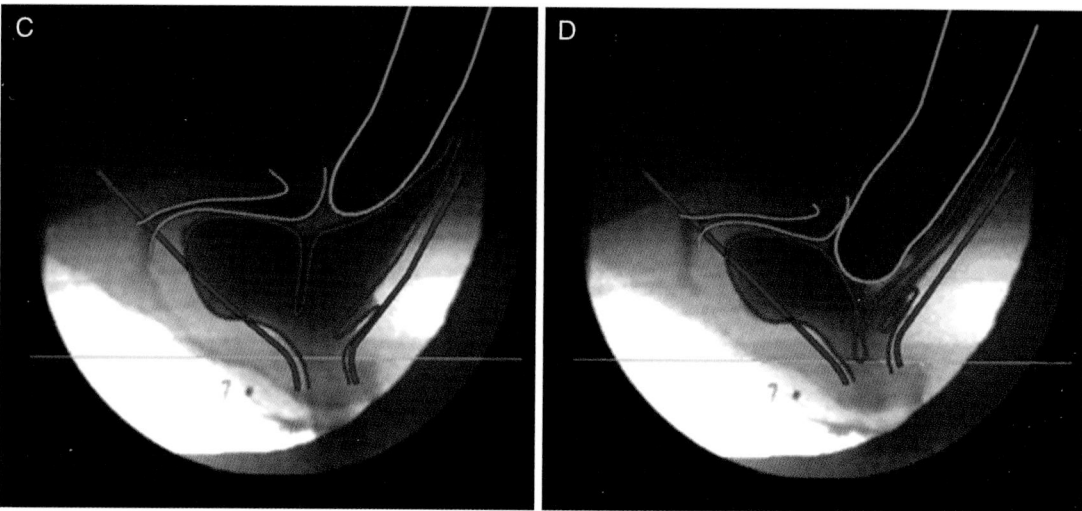

FIG. 1.5. (continued) Defecating proctography illustrating the characteristic anatomical abnormalities associated with ODS. (**a**) as the patient begins to strain an anterior rectocele begins to appear; (**b**) the vagina assumes a horizontal position, the rectocele enlarges, and a small intussusception becomes apparent, (**c**) the internal rectal prolapse (intussusception) increases and descends toward the anal canal, (**d**) the internal rectal prolapse plugs the anal canal, the rectocele fails to empty, and complete obstruction to defecation results

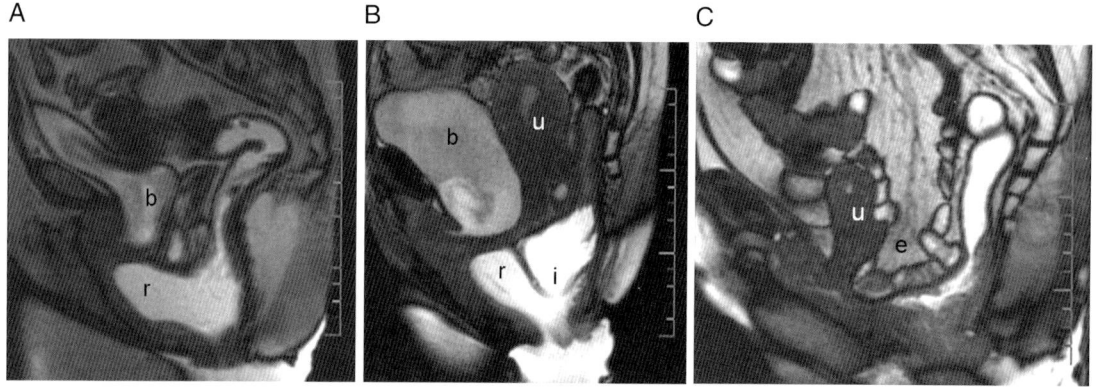

FIG. 1.6. Dynamic MRI images illustrating the characteristic anatomical abnormalities associated with ODS. (**a**) formation of a large anterior rectocele, (**b**) the vagina assumes a horizontal position, and the rectum evaginates as a rectocele and invaginates as an internal rectal prolapse, (**c**) an enterocele descends to fill a low-lying Pouch of Douglas, obstructing defecation. *b* bladder, *r* rectum, *i* internal rectal prolapse (intussusception), *u* uterus, *e* enterocele

Patients suffering from ODS symptoms invariably demonstrate a distal rectal prolapse, which may be isolated or associated with genital prolapse. It is the prolapse which is responsible for fecal obstruction. Compensatory mechanisms may exist to counteract the effects of the prolapse as previously described. In the early stages such compensatory mechanisms may involve the rectum alone, but as the disorder progresses extrarectal anatomical alterations are observed with deepening of the Pouch of Douglas and the formation of enteroceles, sigmoidoceles, and perineal descent in an attempt to facilitate rectal emptying. In later stages, these mechanisms are no longer able to overcome the obstruction exerted by the internal prolapse/intussusception, and defecation can only be achieved by the use of external aids in the form of enemas, laxatives, or Digitations.

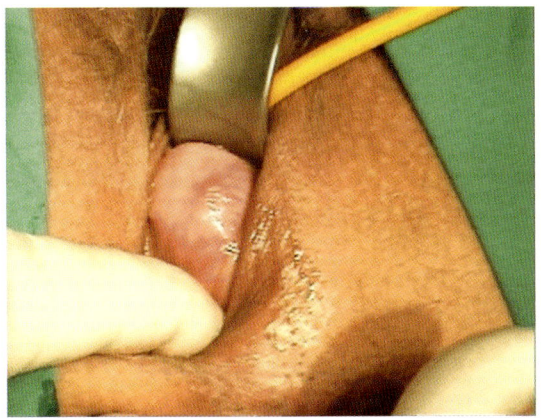

Fig. 1.7. Intraoperative appearance of a rectocele. The examining finger in the rectum bulges forward into the lower vagina

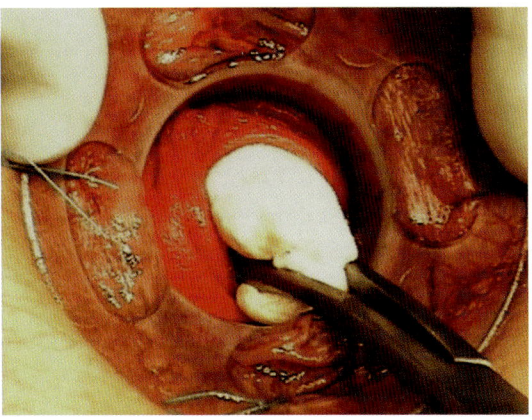

Fig. 1.8. Intraoperative demonstration of internal rectal prolapse. The circular anal dilator of the PPH01 set is placed in the anal canal. A dry swab on a sponge holder is inserted and slowly withdrawn, bringing with it the prolapsing distal rectum

The Development of Stapled Transanal Rectal Resection

It was noted that in patients treated with stapled hemorrhoidopexy, who also had symptoms of outlet obstruction, there was an improvement in not just the hemorrhoidal symptoms but also in rectal evacuatory function. This observation spurred further investigations into the role of distal rectal redundancy as the cause of obstructed defecation, and its possible treatment by transanal stapled resection. A novel surgical treatment for ODS was thus conceived: the Stapled TransAnal Rectal Resection (STARR). This aimed to resect the redundant distal rectum in patients with rectocele/intussusception with restoration of the normal rectal anatomy and relief of symptoms.

The challenge was to produce a full-thickness, transanal, rectal resection incorporating the distal rectal redundancy. A stapling approach was preferred as it avoided opening of the extrarectal spaces, and could achieve simultaneous resection and anastomosis with better control of hemostasis. Such an approach had never before been used for the treatment of ODS.

The initial solution to this problem was to modify the technique of stapled hemorrhoidopexy, utilizing the same PPH 33 mm stapler, but to use two staplers to achieve separate anterior and posterior full-thickness rectal resections with the staple lines meeting on the lateral rectal walls, the so-called PPH-STARR technique. Preliminary results were encouraging, and during the years 1999–2006 the technique increased in popularity, initially in Italy and then across Europe. Several studies, albeit mostly of personal series, were published supporting the short-term efficacy and safety of the technique. This was accompanied by concerns regarding potential complications, the reliability of the technique in the long term, and the need for further evaluation and research (see Chap. 8). In April 2006, the National Institute for Health and Clinical Excellence (NICE) in the UK issued its guidance on the STARR procedure. It noted a lack of good evidence on which to base recommendations and concluded that STARR should only be undertaken if arrangements were in place for audit and review of outcomes. In response to this Italy, Germany, and the UK set up national Registries regulated by their national coloproctology societies, to collect as much data as possible on patients undergoing STARR. The individual Registries were deliberately designed such that the data could be merged into a single STARR Registry (see Chap. 9). The findings of this Registry will be invaluable in guiding future recommendations regarding the application of STARR.

Despite the initial encouraging results from PPH-STARR, the technique does suffer from some inherent drawbacks. The procedure attempts to produce a circumferential full-thickness rectal resection, but has to achieve this with the use of two stapled resections, one placed anteriorly and the other posteriorly. The resulting resection as a consequence is often not uniformly equal around the entire circumference, with a tendency to less tissue being resected at the lateral margins. The resection is performed in a blinded fashion in that it is not possible to predetermine the extent of the prolapse to be resected, which is purely dictated by the housing capacity of the stapler. This housing capacity is limited, and in cases of large internal prolapse may be inadequate for optimal tissue resection. Moreover, potentially serious complications have been reported as a consequence of improper application of the technique [69].

In an attempt to resolve some of the inherent limitations of the PPH-STARR procedure, a new transanal stapler, the Contour Transtar (STR5G), was designed specifically for the purpose. This device is smaller version of the Contour-40 stapler used in anterior resection. Like the Contour-40, it is a curved stapler but with a 30-mm diameter. It is reloadable for multiple stapler firings and incorporates a knife for simultaneous anastomosis and resection. The Contour Transtar comes packaged in a dedicated kit, which includes a circular anal dilator and anoscope. Experience with the new Contour Transtar is to date very preliminary and based purely on personal experience, but it would appear that the results are at least as good as the PPH-STARR technique. Whether the advantages of Contour Transtar in terms of improved operative visualization, adaptable depth of resection, and true circumferential resection translate into improved clinical outcomes remains to be seen. A full description of PPH-STARR and Contour Transtar is included in Chap. 7.

Summary

It has taken over a decade for stapled hemorrhoidopexy to become established as an alternative to conventional hemorrhoidectomy for the treatment of prolapsing piles. Even today, the technique has its opponents, who remain unconvinced regarding its safety and long-term efficacy. However, stapled hemorrhoidopexy is here to stay, and it remains to be seen whether or not it will eventually replace conventional hemorrhoidectomy as the "gold standard."

It is likely that a similar length of time will be required before STARR is accepted as a recognized treatment for obstructed defecation. However, STARR has the advantage in that lessons have been learnt from the introduction of stapled hemorrhoidopexy. As a result, the dissemination of STARR among the surgical community has been more controlled with mechanisms in place for auditing of outcomes. It remains to be seen where STARR will eventually feature in the array of surgical approaches that are available for the treatment of pelvic floor dysfunction.

References

1. Abcarian H, Alexander-Williams J, Christiansen J, Johanson JF, Killingback M, Nelson RL, et al.. Benign anorectal disease: definition, characterization and analysis of treatment. Am J Gastroenterol 1994; 89: S182–S193
2. Johanson JF, Sonnenberg A. The prevalence of hemorrhoids and chronic constipation. An epidemiologic study. Gastroenterology 1990; 98: 380–386
3. Gazet JC, Redding W, Rickett JWS. The prevalence of haemorrhoids. Proc R Soc Med 1970; 63: 78
4. Stapled haemorrhoidopexy for the treatment of haemorrhoids. NICE technology appraisal guidance 128. Available at www.http://nice.org.uk/TA128
5. Johanson JF, Sonneberg A. Temporal changes in the occurrence of haemorrhoids in the United States and England. Dis Colon Rectum 1991; 34: 585
6. Loder PB, Kamm MA, Nicholls RJ. Haemorrhoids: pathology, pathophysiology and aetiology. Br J Surg 1994; 81: 946
7. Bleday R, Pena JP, Rothenberger DA, Goldberg SM, Buls JG. Symptomatic hemorrhoids: current incidence and complications of operative surgery. Dis Colon Rectum 1992; 35: 477–481
8. Whitehead W. Three hundred cases of haemorrhoids cured by excision. Br Med J 1887; 1: 449
9. Milligan ETC, Morgan CN, Jones LE, Officer R. Surgical anatomy of the anal canal and operative treatment of hemorrhoids. Lancet 1937; 2: 1119–1124
10. Parks AG. The surgical treatment of haemorrhoids. Br J Surg 1956; 43: 337–351
11. Fergusson JA, Heaton JR. Closed haemorrhoidectomy. Dis Colon Rectum 1959; 2: 176–179
12. Sharif HI, Lee L, Alexander-Williams J. Diathermy haemorrhoidectomy. Int J Colorectal Dis 1991; 6: 217

Chapter 2
Anatomy and Physiology of Anorectal Prolapse

S.R. Brown and A.J. Shorthouse

Abstract The pathophysiology of hemorrhoids and obstructed defecation requires a sound knowledge of the structure and function of the pelvic floor. The essential structure of this area is discussed with a specific emphasis on applied anatomy. Current theories regarding the physiology of continence and defecation are described. These concepts are then applied to explain the underlying pathophysiology of hemorrhoids and obstructed defecation.

Introduction

Anatomy and physiology sections of medical textbooks are generally dismissed as rather dull and largely unnecessary starters to the main course of sought-after clinical material. However, knowledge of the anatomy and physiology of the anorectum is crucial to understanding how normal continence is maintained, the mechanisms of defecation, and the concepts underpinning the evolution of stapling techniques described later in this book.

This chapter is deliberately selective in concentrating on those aspects of applied anatomy and pathophysiology which are relevant to the stapling procedures used in the treatment of hemorrhoids, anorectal prolapse, and obstructed defecation syndrome (ODS).

Essential Anatomy

Anal Canal

The anal canal extends posteroinferiorly from the lower extremity of the rectum to the anus. It is normally 2–4 cm in length, and its superior part lies in the pelvic cavity. It is surrounded by the internal anal sphincter, which is the thickened inferior extension of the circular muscle of the rectum, and longitudinal muscle fibers derived from the longitudinal rectal muscle coat. The levator muscles condense around the uppermost anal canal to form the puborectalis sling. Inferiorly, the puborectalisfuses with the deep external sphincter, which is contiguous with the superficial external anal sphincter below. These voluntary muscles surround and enclose the internal sphincter and anal epithelium in a cylindrical fashion, but are separated from them by the intersphincteric space, which is a largely avascular anatomic plane of areolar tissue, containing a series of anal glands, and also longitudinal muscle fibers. The inferior part of the anal canal lies in the perineum and is surrounded by the superficial part of the external sphincter which, together with fibers of the longitudinal muscle, is responsible for forming radial corrugations at the point of attachment to the perianal skin (Fig. 2.1).

It is important to clarify definitions. The anatomic anal canal is defined as the region from the dentate

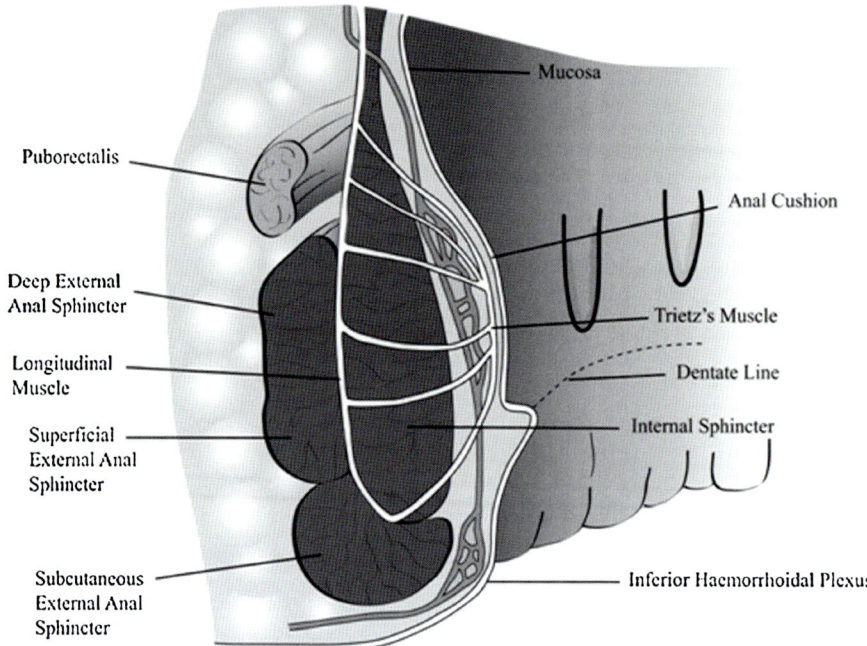

FIG. 2.1. Anatomy of the anal canal with particular reference to the structure of the anal cushions. Fibroelastic and muscular tissues form a scaffold that supports the vascular infrastructure of the cushions. Contraction leads to compression of the vascular anal cushions, increasing the luminal diameter of the anal canal and aiding evacuation. Rupture of the supporting scaffold results in prolapse of the cushions, failure of adequate compression during evacuation, and subsequent engorgement of the vascular component. Note also the fibers from the superficial external sphincter and the longitudinal muscle inserting into the perianal skin to form the anal skin corrugations

line to the anal verge, in contrast to the surgical anal canal which is the area extending from the anorectal junction to the anal verge.

Rectum

The junction of the sigmoid colon and rectum has always been a matter of debate between surgeons and anatomists. Although its distinction is of importance in rectal cancer surgery, the upper extent of the rectum is of limited relevance in the treatment of anorectal prolapse. A description of the lower rectum is highly relevant: its distal end is limited by the upper end of the anal canal, where the anorectal angle is directed posteriorly as it passes through the pelvic floor. This corresponds to the level of the puborectalis muscle. Active contraction of this muscle maintains the angle between the rectum and the anal canal, acting as a sling to pull the anorectal angle forward, and is the most important component of the continence mechanism (Fig. 2.2).

The rectum may be arbitrarily divided into three regions related to its coverings: the upper rectum is covered in peritoneum anteriorly and laterally, the middle third only anteriorly, and the lower third is devoid of a covering as the peritoneum is reflected forward onto the seminal vesicles and bladder in the male and vagina and uterus in the female. This forms a pocket of peritoneum, the pouch of Douglas, which is variable in its extent. The peritoneal reflection lies approximately 8 cm from the perineal skin in men and 5–8 cm in women. It is particularly deep in patients with a full-thickness rectal prolapse and in those patients with an enterocoele or sigmoidocoele. It is important to be aware of this when carrying out full-thickness rectal stapling techniques as incorporation of the peritoneum into the staple line increases the risk of small bowel or sigmoid colon being included in the staple line. Inclusion of the peritoneal lining in the staple line also carries a risk of peritonitis in the event of staple line dehiscence, when the rectal lumen will communicate directly with the pelvic cavity.

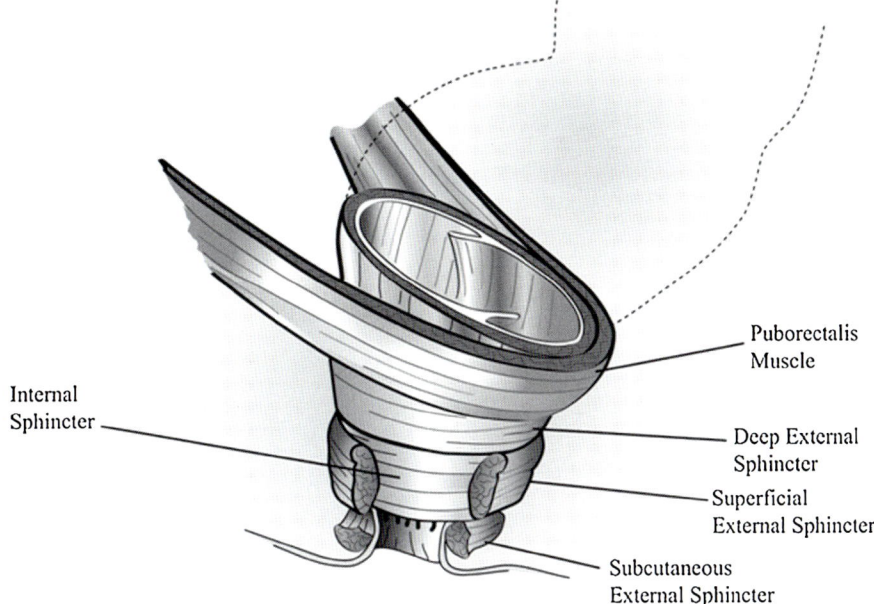

Internal
Sphincter

Puborectalis
Muscle

Deep External
Sphincter

Superficial
External Sphincter

Subcutaneous
External Sphincter

Fig. 2.2. Components of the anal sphincter. The puborectalis acts as a sling to pull the anorectal junction forward. This plays an important role in maintaining continence

A discrete layer of dense connective tissue, comprising collagen, smooth muscle, and elastin fibers, can be found between the rectum and the vagina, and has been well demonstrated by operative and cadaveric studies [1, 2]. The rectovaginal fascia extends from the cervix to the perineum, merging laterally into the fascial covering of the iliococcygeus and pubococcygeus muscles. It provides support for the rectal wall and, in the normal female, resists the effect of increased intra-abdominal pressure to form an anterior rectocele.

Posteriorly the rectum follows the curve of the sacrum, and as it passes downward and forward to meet the anal canal, it angulates sharply backward and inferiorly. This has significance for purse string insertion during stapling procedures, as there is a tendency to spiral the suture downward posteriorly, risking incorporation of part of the puborectalis muscle into the staple line. This may be a potential cause of postoperative pain.

Arterial and Venous Drainage

Anatomical descriptions of the arterial supply to the rectum and anal canal generally list five main arteries, which anastomose together to a variable extent.

Three of these arteries are usually encountered in various forms during mesorectal dissection. The inferior mesenteric artery continues as the superior rectal artery when it reaches the pelvic brim, and is the most consistent of these arteries, dividing into right and left branches at the level of S3. Two midrectal arteries (arising from the internal iliac arteries) are less consistent [3–5]. Two inferior rectal arteries are encountered in abdominoperineal resection, as they arise from the internal pudendal arteries high in the ischiorectal fossa.

A rich venous plexus surrounds the surface of the rectum in the submucosal plane and is relevant to stapling techniques. The plexus drains into the superior, middle, and inferior rectal veins, which follow the course of the arteries (Fig. 2.3). This is a well-known example of a portosystemic communication: the superior rectal vein drains into the portal system, whereas the middle and the inferior rectal veins enter the systemic system via the internal iliac veins. There is a free communication with other pelvic plexuses which explains an increased predisposition for engorgement and other hemorrhoidal symptoms in situations of increased pelvic blood flow, for example during pregnancy and, to a lesser extent, menstruation.

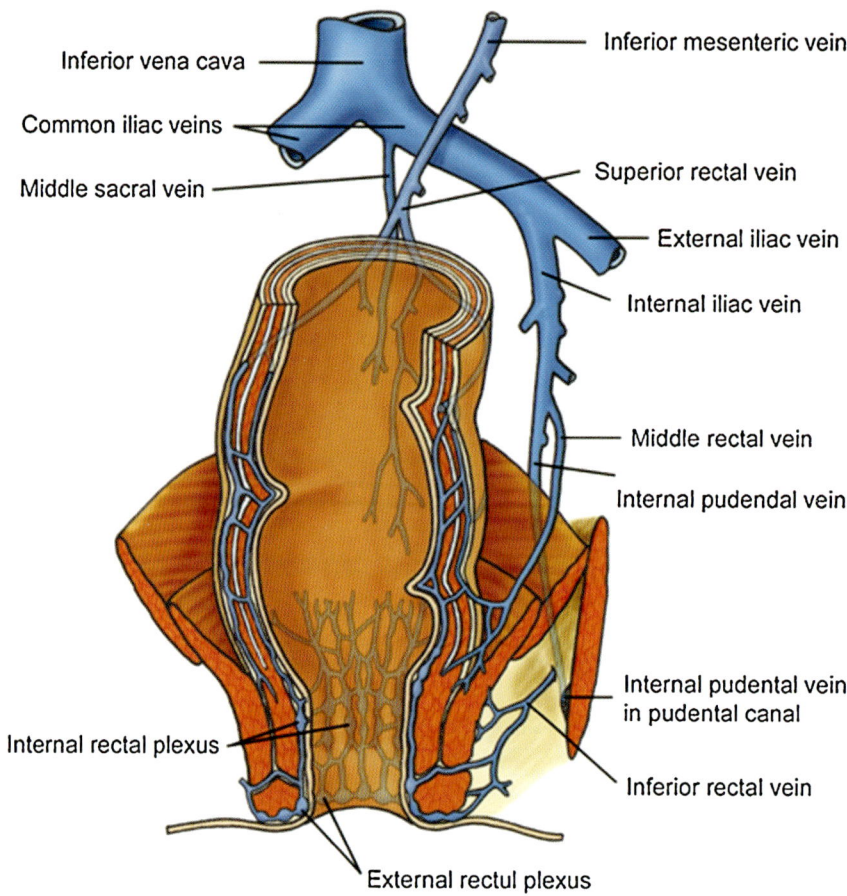

Inferior vena cava

Common iliac veins

Middle sacral vein

Inferior mesenteric vein

Superior rectal vein

External iliac vein

Internal iliac vein

Middle rectal vein

Internal pudendal vein

Internal pudental vein
in pudental canal

Inferior rectal vein

Internal rectal plexus

External rectul plexus

FIG. 2.3. Venous drainage of the rectum and anal canal. Note the rich venous submucosal plexus. Note also the drainage into portal and systemic systems and free communication with genital and visceral plexuses

Epithelial Lining

Skin extends into the distal anal canal as far as the lower border of the internal anal sphincter, and is lined by stratified squamous keratinizing epithelium, with sweat glands, hair follicles, and sebaceous glands. Stratified nonkeratinizing squamous epithelium extends from this level to the dentate line and is devoid of these structures. Immediately above the dentate line is the anal transition zone (ATZ), which is a layer of mixed stratified and columnar epithelium approximately 1 cm in length. The ATZ is important for anal sampling and the maintenance of continence (see later).

At the dentate line is a series of approximately twelve papillae, which sometimes enlarge and fibrose in response to anal fissures or hemorrhoidal

complications, such as thrombosis. Anal glands drain into a series of ducts lined by squamous epithelium, and which cross the internal sphincter to open at the dentate line behind the papillae. These are thought to predispose to anal sepsis and fistula formation [6].

Longitudinal mucosal columns, usually situated in the left lateral, right posterior, and right anterior aspects of the upper anal canal and ending at the dentate line, arise from the anal cushions above.

Microstructure of the Anal Cushions

The elegant anatomical injection studies of Thomson demonstrated the structure and function of the anal cushions [4]. All the arteries to the rectum supply the hemorrhoidal cushions. The cushions consist of a fibroelastic and muscular network within vascular lakes, which drain directly into the superior, middle, and inferior rectal veins at various levels within the confines of the anal sphincters. Uniquely, there is no intervening capillary network. Radiological and serial section histological techniques have shown that arteriovenous channels communicate directly with the venous lakes via a system of arterioles passing through the muscle wall of the distal rectum. This explains why hemorrhoidal bleeding is bright red. These complex channels, interlaced by a fibroelastic and muscular network derived from the longitudinal part of the internal sphincter (Fig. 2.1), function as a scaffold, providing architectural support for the cushions. The scaffold concept was originally described by Trietz more than 150 years ago.

Anal Sphincters, Pelvic Floor Muscles, and Ligaments

The circular muscle coat of the rectum extends and thickens as it enters the anal canal to form the internal anal sphincter. It ends as a well-defined palpable rounded edge immediately superior to the anal margin.

The longitudinal muscle of the rectum blends with pubococcygeus at the anorectal junction, but some fibers continue downward in the intersphincteric space and, diverging beyond the lower border of the external anal sphincter, attach to the skin of the perianal region to function as an anchor.

The external sphincter, puborectalis, and levator animaintain voluntary continence. Levator ani is a muscular diaphragm and supports the pelvic floor. It consists of a cradle-like sheet of muscle (the levator plate), which arises from various bony prominences around the pelvis, and is deficient in the midline where the pelvic viscera pass through. The perineal bodyand anococcygeal ligament lie anterior and posterior to the anal canal, respectively, to form insertions for levator ani, transverse perineii, and the external anal sphincter. These condensations anchor the anal canal to the pelvic bones (Fig. 2.4).

Levator ani has four component parts, of which puborectalis is the most prominent, forming a sling around the anorectal junction and contiguous with the external sphincter as a functioning unit for maintenance of continence.

There are three levels of support for the vagina [7, 8]:

1. The cardinal-uterosacral complex supports the cervix and vagina above the levator plate.
2. Lateral connections to the arcus tendinous fascia of the pelvis support the midvagina.
3. Connections to the perineal membrane anteriorly and the perineal body posteriorly also support the mid vagina.

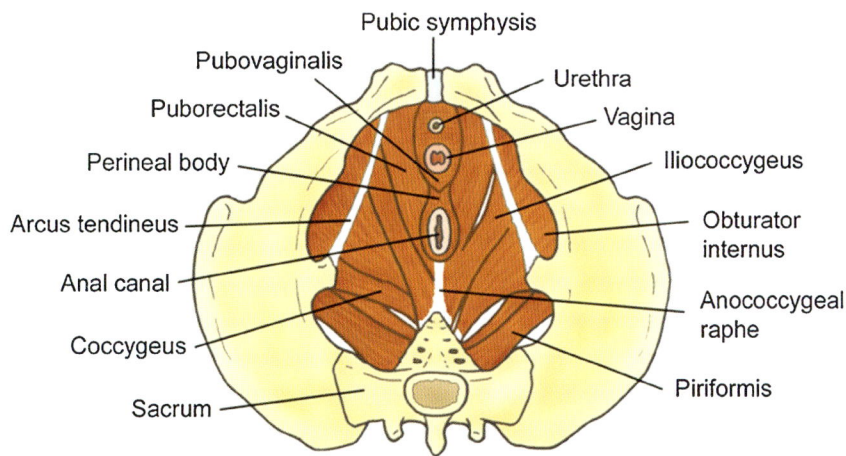

Pubic symphysis
Pubovaginalis
Puborectalis
Perineal body
Arcus tendineus
Anal canal
Coccygeus
Sacrum
Urethra
Vagina
Iliococcygeus
Obturator internus
Anococcygeal raphe
Piriformis

FIG. 2.4. Structure of the pelvic diaphragm. The perineal body is formed by fusion of the levator ani, transverse perineii, and the external sphincter muscles. Together with the anococcygeal ligament, they act as anchors to give the funnel shape of the pelvic diaphragm

Nerve Supply

Sympathetic and Parasympathetic Innervation

The anorectum and the pelvic floor are supplied by sympathetic, parasympathetic, and somatic nerve fibers. Sympathetic innervation is derived from the sympathetic trunk via the superior hypogastric nerve plexus. Parasympathetic fibers originate from ventral rami of the second, third, and often the fourth sacral nerves (S2–4). Sacral parasympathetic pathways to the colon have excitatory and inhibitory components [9]. Excitatory pathways play an important role in colonic propulsive activity, especially during defecation. Inhibitory pathways allow colonic volume to adapt to its contents, and also mediate descending inhibition, which initiates colonic relaxation ahead of a fecal bolus.

Somatic Innervation

Somatic branches travel mainly in the pudendal nerve to supply motor fibers, mainly voluntary, to the external anal sphincter and levator ani, and also sensory fibers to the anus.

Anorectal Sensation

Modalities of anal sensation can be precisely defined [10]. The anal canal is extremely sensitive to touch, pain, temperature, and movement. For many of these stimuli, sensitivity is greater than that of the perianal skin, which has a similar level of sensitivity to the dorsum of the hand. Sensory perception varies throughout the anal canal and is maximal within the ATZ. Above the ATZ, sensation is similar to that within the rectum.. Potentially painful stimuli, such as band ligation or PPH, must therefore be carried out well above the upper limit of the ATZ. This upper limit can be very variable.

In contrast to anal sensation, certain modalities of rectal sensation are indistinct. The rectum is insensitive to stimuli such as pain or touch, but sensitive to distension. Distension of a rectal balloon gives a sensation of the need to defecate particularly in the ampulla. The course of the sensory fibers detecting distension is unclear, but they probably pass through the inferior hypogastric plexus to the spinal cord and are responsible for the rectoanal inhibitory reflex. Evidence from patients who have undergone rectal excision and coloanal anastomosis but who still have sensation to distension suggests that nerve endings are present in the surrounding pelvic floor structures [11]. Indistinct rectal sensation for pain allows surgery in this area to be carried out without the type of acute postoperative pain normally experienced after surgery below the dentate line. However, patients do sometimes experience aching pelvic pain after procedures such as banding and stapled hemorrhoidopexy (PPH), even when the intervention has been carried out well above the dentate line [12–14]. The etiology of this pain is unclear. Following band ligation, any pain appears to be related to the number of bands placed, is seldom severe, and often resolves within 24–48 h [12]. Persistent pain after PPH is uncommon but, in the absence of any other cause, may be related to sphincter spasm [14].

The rectoanal inhibitory reflex occurs when the internal anal sphincter relaxes almost immediately after distension of the rectum, and is dependent on mechanoreceptors in the rectum but independent of higher center control. Duthie and Bennett suggested that internal sphincter relaxation allows rectal contents to be "sampled" by the sensitive anal transition zone and the lower anal canal [15]. Sampling allows discrimination between feces and flatus and appears to be an important component of continence [16].

Physiology of Defecation

Maintenance of Continence

During the resting phase, the high-pressure zone in the anal canal can maintain continence, even when the rectum is full. Resting pressure results mainly from internal anal sphincter tone, but there is a 15–20% contribution from the external sphincter [17, 18] and up to 15% from the anal cushions [19–22]. The cushions act as a seal to create a watertight anal canal and function as a unit with the sphincters: without them the internal sphincter would lose much of its tone, as it needs the arteriolar pressure within the cushions to generate its resting pressure, until the two reach a state of tonic equilibrium at rest. A mucinous film covering the sealed cushions completes the seal by means of surface tension. Hemorrhoidal prolapse reduces the efficiency of the seal, due to reduced resting pressure, allowing seepage [23]. Similarly, excision of the anal cushions during hemorrhoidectomy will result in reduced efficiency of the seal which, together with the effects of scarring and deformity, may lead to postoperative soiling.

Although the external sphincter is in a state of tonic contraction and contributes to resting tone, its main function is voluntary contraction. Under central control, it maintains continence when it is socially inappropriate to defecate after initiation of the rectoanal inhibitory reflex. It also contracts as part of a reflex in unison with the other striated muscles of the pelvic floor to maintain continence during coughing, straining, or other instances of sudden rises in intra-abdominal pressure.

Other factors influencing continence include rectal filling and compliance. As the rectum fills, it relaxes to maintain a fairly constant intrarectal pressure, until a compliance threshold is reached after which any further rise in pressure results in a desire to defecate. Progressive reduction in compliance results in urgency and eventually frank incontinence. Loss of sensation to rectal filling, as seen in cases of pudendal neuropathy or cauda equina lesions, leads to incontinence when rectal pressure exceeds anal pressure, and before the subject is even aware of the need to defecate.

Stool consistency and volume are also important for continence. Small pellet stools are more difficult to expel than large deformable stools. In addition pellet stools are more likely to result in soiling due to difficulty in evacuating completely. Small hard pellets accumulate in the rectum causing abdominal distension and sometimes incontinence, without even stimulating the urge to defecate [24]. Bulking agents avoid pellet stool formation and enable stool to be evacuated from the rectum more easily. Liquid stool is more likely to lead to incontinence, even in the normal subject. Rectal hypersensitivity is also associated with fecal incontinence and aggravated by loose stool, for instance in irritable bowel syndrome. In inflammatory bowel disease incontinence results from a combination of hypersensitivity, diarrhea, and loss of rectal compliance.

Defecation

Rectal distension produces a sensation of rectal fullness [25] and is probably mediated through receptors in the pelvic floor muscles, as it remains after coloanal anastomosis [10, 26]. Distension triggers the rectoanal inhibitory reflex, which permits sampling of rectal contents by the nerve-rich ATZ of the anal canal and allows discrimination between feces and flatus. Reflex contraction of the external sphincter maintains continence. Two examples of the importance of the rectoanal inhibitory reflex in maintaining continence are given. Firstly reduced continence is seen in some patients after low anterior resection when the reflex may be lost [27]. Secondly some surgical procedures which restore the ATZ from a prolapsed state into a more correct anatomical position (e.g., sphincter repair and rectopexy) have been shown to restore continence by improving anal sensation [28, 29]. This second example may also apply to stapled hemorrhoidopexy.

When the internal sphincter relaxes there is a conscious desire to defecate and evacuation occurs, unless the call to stool is inconvenient. As the external sphincter relaxes, stool evacuates and is helped by voluntarily increasing intra-abdominal pressure. Squatting increases the anorectal angle and produces more efficient stool transmission. Completion of defecation is achieved by a closing reflex, when the external anal sphincter contracts and propels residual fecal material back into the rectum leaving an empty anal canal [20].

An understanding of the microstructure of the anal cushion sex plains their role in maintaining continence and aiding evacuation. Abundant venous drainage channels allow passive compression and widening of the anal canal as stool passes through the relaxed internal sphincter. Contraction of the fibroelastic muscle also actively compresses the venous dilatations. Finally, alteration in shape and eversion of the cushions aid evacuation as stool passes through (Fig. 2.5).

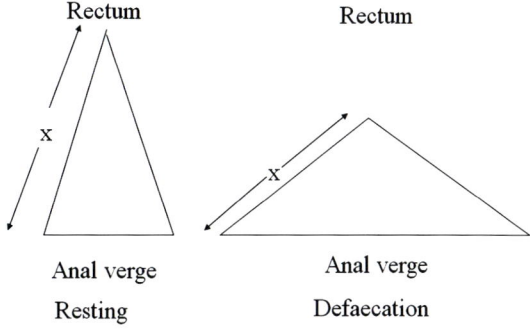

FIG. 2.5. Diagrammatic illustration of how the altered position and the form of the anal cushions aid evacuation. The length of the anal cushions (x) remains constant during defecation. However, the lumen of the anal canal dilates by relaxation of the internal and external sphincters and increased tension in anal cushion fibroelastic microstructure, resulting in venous lake compression. Consequently the cushions shorten and stool expulsion is augmented

Pathophysiology of Hemorrhoids

The anal cushions play a significant role in maintaining continence and facilitating evacuation. The term "hemorrhoids" should only be used if there is change in cushion morphology or function, resulting in hemorrhoidal symptoms such as prolapse, fresh bleeding, seepage, perianal irritation, or thrombosis.

There are many theories about the evolution of hemorrhoids [4]. Portal hypertension and varicose veins have been discounted by detailed anatomical and histological studies, demonstrating that venous dilations are integral to normal anal cushion structure. Patients with portal hypertension have a higher incidence of anorectal varices, but these are an entirely distinct anatomical and clinical entity. In fact, hemorrhoids per se are seen less frequently in patients with portal hypertension than in the general population. Recurrent infection of the anal lining has also been proposed as a cause of hemorrhoids but is untenable as the anal canal is very resistant to infection due to its excellent blood supply.

Epidemiology plays an important role in the etiology of hemorrhoids, which occur less commonly in geographical areas where diet is rich in fiber [30]. Harder, drier pellet stools, or large fecal masses result in straining with obstructed venous return and engorgement. However, the prevalence of constipation does not correlate particularly well with the occurrence of hemorrhoids, as many with the condition have a normal bowel habit.

The sliding mucosa theory [4] proposes that hemorrhoids arise from degeneration of Trietz's muscle, the fibromuscular scaffold forming the supporting tissue of the anal cushions. The cushions prolapse and engorge due to interruption of venous return and pressure from the anal canal, with the potential to precipitate thrombosis.

The following observations support the sliding mucosa theory:

1. Anal cushions are present in both the asymptomatic individual and fetus. Their structure is similar to that found in patients with symptomatic hemorrhoids [4].
2. Smooth muscle is often noted in excisional specimens.
3. Fiber-poor diet and straining are likely to result in degeneration and rupture of Trietz's muscle, making prolapse more likely.
4. A genetic predisposition to hemorrhoids can be explained by the presence of an inherited connective tissue weakness, perhaps also explaining the association of hemorrhoids with genital prolapse and hernias.
5. Aging is associated with fragmentation of the fibromuscular scaffold and correlates with an increase in hemorrhoidal symptoms.
6. Outpatient hemorrhoidal treatments, such as injection sclerotherapy, infrared coagulation, or elastic band ligation, fix the mucosa to the underlying rectal muscle wall, with restoration of the function of the suspensory muscle of Trietz.
7. Hemorrhoids resolve after abdominal rectopexy for rectal prolapse.

The rationale for stapled hemorrhoidopexy fits well with the sliding mucosa theory, as it aims to restore the prolapsed "hemorrhoids" to their original anatomical position. It restores anal cushion function by correcting anal sphincter pressure above the prolapse and reducing the submucosal arterial supply from the rectum. The level of the stapled anastomosis is placed well above the upper limit of somatic pain sensation within the anal canal, and is the reason for reduced postoperative pain and more rapid recovery after stapled hemorrhoidopexy as compared with excisional hemorrhoidectomy.

Pathophysiology of ODS

Normal defecation requires normal colonic transit, intact anorectal sensation, appropriate expulsion forces and coordinated pelvic floor function. Disturbance of any of these factors can lead to constipation. Obstructed defecation syndrome(ODS) arises when pelvic floor dysfunction results in an impaired ability to satisfactorily evacuate the rectum. The diagnosis should only be made after other organic causes, such as tumor or stenosis, having been excluded.

Different causes of ODS are listed in Table 2.1 [31] and discussed in more detail.

TABLE 2.1. Mechanisms of ODS and associated disorders.

Causes of ODS	Examples
Diminished rectal sensation	Megarectum
	Large rectocele
	Cauda equina lesion
	Pudendal neuropathy
	Diabetes mellitus
	Demyelinating neurological disease
Functional outlet obstruction	Hirshsprung's disease
	Chagas' disease
Failure to relax IAS	Anismus
Failure to relax pelvic floor	Spinal cord lesions
	Multiple Sclerosis
Mechanical outlet obstruction	Intussusception
	Full-thickness rectal prolapse
	Enterocele or sigmoidocele
	Uterine descent
Inefficient force vector	Rectocele
	Descending perineum
	Full-thickness rectal prolapse

Diminished Rectal Sensitivity

Sensory awareness of the presence of feces in the rectum is necessary to initiate the rectoanal inhibitory reflex and the sampling reflex. Whether or not defecation follows depends on central mechanisms and the conscious desire to defecate. Hyposensitivity occurs when the rectum is too large and more compliant, with raised sensory thresholds, or when there is a defect in the receptor or neural pathways. Both result in failure to initiate defecation.

Failure to Relax the Internal Sphincter

Relaxation of the internal sphincter is essential for evacuation to occur. Relaxation is coordinated via the sympathetic trunk and interruption of any part of the reflex pathway will result in constipation.

Failure to Relax the Pelvic Floor

A spastic pelvic floor will also result in difficulty in evacuation. In this group anismus (anal dysynergia, spastic pelvic floor syndrome, puborectalis syndrome or paradox) deserves specific mention. It is defined as an increase in anal pressure during attempted defecation in conjunction with an impairment of rectal emptying and is a functional disorder characteristically seen in younger women, who often have normal anatomy.

It is thought to be due to abnormal rectoanal coordination with inappropriate contraction of the puborectalis and external anal sphincter muscles during straining [32, 33] Precise definition of the condition is difficult, as anorectal manometry, electrophysiology, and dynamic proctography may show the same abnormalities in patients with other conditions or normal individuals without obstructed defecation [34–36]. In some cases a finding of puborectalis paradox may be artifactual, due to defecation being attempted under nonphysiological laboratory conditions [37]. Defecation is a learned behavioral response, and habitual events that invoke altered behavior, such as anxiety, may be sufficient to change colonic and pelvic floor function. Paradoxical contractions are more likely to be representative of inappropriate defecation behavior rather than a true underlying pathology, with anismus being part of a more complex derangement of higher center control. Behavioral therapy (biofeedback) is an appropriate therapeutic strategy in these patients.

Mechanical Outlet Obstruction

Another prerequisite for effective evacuation is a clear channel for stool to progress from the rectum through the anal canal. Anal strictures or stenosing rectal cancers are obvious organic causes of obstruction. Other anorectal abnormalities such as intussusception may be associated with obstructed defecation, although even large intussusceptions may sometimes cause no symptoms at all. Extrinsic obstruction can result from straining in the presence of an enterocele or sigmoidocele within in a deep pouch of Douglas, when defecation can become difficult to initiate and complete [38]. An enlarged uterus can produce a similar effect.

Inefficient Force Vector

Increased intra-abdominal pressure forcefully expels rectal contents and is often necessary for successful evacuation. However, it requires channeling of the force that increases intrarectal pressure, which in turn is dependent on a degree of resistance from the supporting structures of the rectum and pelvis. A "loss of push" occurs if the force is dissipated by bulging of the rectum forward (rectocele), or downward (intussusception and descending perineum).

Rectocele

A rectocele is a type of pelvic organ prolapse in which there is herniation of the posterior vaginal wall forward, with the anterior attenuated rectal wall in direct contact with the vagina. Straining results in bulging of the rectocele at the expense of efficient evacuation, and stool is more likely to be directed into the rectocele rather than the anal canal. This is not always the case, as sometimes a normal defecation pattern is found in the presence of even a large rectocele

There are various levels of support for the vagina and rectum. Defects in any or all will result in a rectocele. A high rectocele is often associated with loss of uterine support and genital prolapse. A rectocele at an intermediate level may be associated with a defect in the rectovaginal septum and causes bulging of the posterior vaginal wall. A low rectocele is often associated with disruption of the perineal body and direct tear from obstetric injury [39]. Childbirth results in stretching and distortion of the pelvic floor, and in some cases disruption of the endopelvic fascia, including the rectovaginal septum and the perineal body. Apart from damage to the supporting structures, another factor predisposing to rectocele development is pudendal neuropathy, caused by stretching, traction, and direct pressure on the pudendal nerve as it traverses the pelvic side wall. This results in partial denervation of the levator ani and sphincter muscles and can occur during childbirth or from long-term straining during defecation.

Both of these changes can progress to perineal descent, widening of the genital hiatus through the levator ani, and generalized perineal laxity, due to degeneration and attenuation of the pelvic floor muscles. Because the vaginal opening can no longer completely close, the posterior vaginal wall is then subjected to an even higher pressure gradient. Similar damage also leads to obstructed defecation, but it is often difficult to distinguish cause and effect, as the anatomical changes themselves perpetuate the need to strain.

Descending Perineum Syndrome

The most prominent symptom of descending perineum syndrome is a permanent and intractable difficulty with evacuation, and is due to injury to the pudendal nerves from trauma, childbirth, or chronic straining to defecate [40, 41]. The perineum bulges on straining, reflecting a lack of pelvic floor support for the rectum and perirectal structures. Not only is there a "loss of push" but the anterior rectal wall also frequently intussuscepts into the anal canal with straining and acts as a plug preventing evacuation [42, 43].

Summary

An understanding of the anatomy and physiology of the pelvic floor, maintenance of fecal continence, and the process of defecation gives some insight not only into the possible mechanisms of system failure but also the underlying principles behind surgical correction. Restoration of normal anatomy and physiology is the ultimate goal if optimal function is to be achieved.

References

1. Richardson AC. The rectovaginal septum revisited: its relationship to rectocele and its importance in rectocele repair. Clin Obstet Gynecol 1993; 36:976–983
2. Milley PS, Nichols DH. A correlative investigation of the human rectovaginal septum. Anat Rec 1969; 163:443–452
3. Jones OM, Smeulders N, Wiseman O, et al. Lateral ligaments of the rectum: an anatomical study. Br J Surg 1999; 86:487–489
4. Thomson WH. The nature of haemorrhoids Br J Surg 1975; 62:542–552
5. Ayoub SF. Arterial supply to the human rectum. Acta Anat Basel 1978; 100:317–327
6. Parks AG. Etiology and surgical treatment of fistula-in-ano. Dis Colon Rect 1963; 6:17–22
7. DeLancey JO. Structural anatomy of the posterior pelvic compartment as it relates to rectocele. Am J Obstet Gynecol 1999; 180:815–823
8. DeLancey JO. Anatomic aspects of vaginal eversion after hysterectomy. Am J Obstet Gynecol 1992; 166:1717–1728
9. Gonella J, Bouvier M, Blanquet F. Extrinsic nervous control of motility of small and large intestines and related sphincters. Physiol Rev 1987; 67:902–961
10. Duthie HL, Gairns FW. Sensory nerve endings and sensation in the anal region in man. Br J Surg 1960; 47:585–595
11. Lane RH, Parks AG. Function of the anal sphincters following colo-anal anastomosis. Br J Surg 1977; 64:596–599

12. Lee HH, Spencer RJ, Beart RW. Multiple haemorrhoidal bandings in a single session. Dis Colon Rect. 1994; 37:37–41

13. Cheetham MJ, Mortensen NJ, Nystrom P-O, Kamm MA, Phillips RK. Persistent pain and faecal urgency after stapled haemorrhoidectomy. Lancet 2000; 356:730–733

14. Thala LA, Irvine LA, Steele RJ, Campbell KL. Postdefaecation pain syndrome after circular stapled anopexy is abolished by oral nifedipine. Br J Surg 2005; 92:208–210

15. Duthie HL, Bennett RC. The relation of sensation in the anal canal to the function of sphincter length: a possible factor in anal incontinence. Gut 1963; 4:179–182

16. Miller R, Bartolo DC, Cervero F, et al. Anorectal sampling: a comparison of normal and incontinent patients. Br J Surg 1988; 75:44–47

17. Duthie HL, Watts J. Contribution of the external anal sphincter to the pressure zone in the anal canal. Gut 1965; 6:64–68

18. Freckner B, von Euler C. Influence of pudendal block on the function of the anal sphincters. Gut 1975; 16:482–489

19. Arabi Y, Alexander-Williams J, Keighley MRB. Anal pressure in haemorrhoids and fissure. Am J Surg 1977; 1:608–610

20. Bennett LRC, Duthie HL. The functional importance of the internal sphincter. Br J Surg 1964; 51:355–357

21. Gibbons CP, Trowbridge EA, Bannister JJ, Read NW. Role of anal cushions in maintaining continence. Lancet 1986; i:886–888

22. Hancock BD, Smith K. The internal anal sphincter and the nature of haemorrhoids. Gut 1977; 18:651–656

23. Schuster MM, Hendrix TR, Mendeloff AI. The internal anal sphincter response: manometric studies on its normal physiology, neural pathways and alteration in bowel disorders. J Clin Invest 1963; 42:196–207

24. Sun WM, Read NW, Shorthouse AJ. Hypertensive anal cushions as a cause of the high anal pressures in patients with haemorrhoids. Br J Surg 1990; 77:458–462

25. Ambrose WL, et-al.. The effect of stool consistency on rectal and neorectal emptying. Dis Colon Rectum 1993; 34:1

26. Winkler G. Remarques sur la morphologie et l'innervation du muscle releur de l'anus. Arch Anat Histol Embryol 1958; 41:77–95

27. Keighley MRB, Yoshioka K, Kmoit W, Heyer F. Physiological parameters influencing functions in restorative proctocolectomy and ileo-pouch-anal anastomosis. Br J Surg 1988; 75:997–1002

28. Lewis WG, Martin IG, Williamson ME, et al. Why do some patients experience poor functional results after anterior resection of the rectum for carcinoma? Dis Colon Rect 1995; 38:259–263

29. Duthie GS, Bartolo DCC. Is improvement of continence after rectopexy for rectal prolapse dependent on improved sphincter function or postoperative constipation? Gut 1989; 30:A1466

30. Burkitt DP, Graham-Stewart CW. Haemorrhoids-postulated pathogenesis and proposed prevention. Postgrad Med J 1975; 51:631–636

31. D'Hoore A, Penninckx F. Obstructed defecation. Colorectal Dis 2003; 5:280–287

32. Kuijpers HC, Bleijenberg G. The spastic pelvic floor yndrome. A cause of constipation. Dis Colon Rect 1985; 28:669–672

33. Kuijpers HC, Bleijenberg G, de Morree H. The spastic pelvic floor syndrome. Large bowel outlet obstruction caused by pelvic floor dysfunction: a radiological study. Int J Colorectal Dis 1986; 1:44–48

34. Jones PN, Lubowski DZ, Swash M & Henry MM. Is paradoxical contraction of puborectalis muscle of functional importance? Dis Colon Rect 1987; 30:667–670

35. Barnes PR, Lennard-Jones JE. Function of the striated anal sphincter during straining in control subjects and constipated patients with a radiologically normal rectum or idiopathic megacolon. Int J Colorectal Dis 1988; 3:207–209

36. Leroi AM, Berkelmans I, Denis P et-al.. Anismus as a marker of sexual abuse. Consequences of abuse on anorectal motility. Dig Dis Sci 1995; 40:1411–1416

37. Duthie GS & Bartolo DC. Anismus: the cause of constipation? Results of investigation and treatment. World J Surg 1992; 16:831–835

38. Holley RL. Enterocele: a review. Obstet Gynecol Surv 1994; 49:284–293

39. Zbar AP, Beer-Gabel M, Aslam M. Rectoanal inhibition and rectocele: physiology versus categorization. Int J Colorectal Dis 2001; 16:307–312

40. Snooks SJ, Setchell M, Swash M. Injury to innervation of pelvic floor sphincter musculature in childbirth. Lancet 1984; 2:546–550

41. Kiff ES, Barnes PB, Henry MM. Prolongation of pudendal nerve latency and increased single fiber density in patients with chronic defecation straining and perineal descent. Br J Surg 1983; 70:681

42. Girona J. Diagnosis and therapeutic possibilities of descending perineum syndrome. Leber Magen Darm. 1992; 22:44–46

43. D'Amico DF, Angriman I. Descending perineum syndrome: iatrogenic or spontaneous pathology? Chir Ital. 2000; 52:625–630

Chapter 3
Diagnosis of Hemorrhoids and ODS

D. Jayne and K.P. Nugent

Abstract Hemorrhoidal disease is a common complaint in the coloproctology outpatient clinic. A careful history and examination is usually all that is required to select patients for surgical intervention. Other investigations are aimed at excluding coexistent colorectal disease and assessing anorectal function in patients with a history of defecatory dysfunction or incontinence. Obstructed defecation may be due to a variety of pathologies. Although a careful history and examination help to define the problem, further investigation of pelvic floor function is mandatory to characterize the underlying etiology. The clinical diagnosis of hemorrhoidal disease and obstructed defecation syndrome is discussed.

Introduction

From the late nineteenth century until the work done by Thomson [1] in 1975, there were three main theories behind the development of symptomatic hemorrhoids. One of the earliest definitions dating from the time of Hippocrates was that hemorrhoids were varicose veins (discrete dilatations of veins) within the anal canal [2]. These dilatations were thought to be pathological, caused either by a localized weakness in the vein wall or a localized increase in venous pressure. The increase in venous pressure was thought to be due to a combination of the portosystemic communication within the anal canal and transmission of increased intra-abdominal pressure during straining [3]. The presence or absence of a communication between the superior rectal vein and the systemic circulation was debated during the nineteenth century [4], but free vascular communications demonstrated by the end of the century suggested that a localized increase in venous pressure was an unlikely cause of hemorrhoids. Indeed, it is likely that the dilated anal canal veins are normal structures as they are seen in asymptomatic children.

The second theory, also popular in the nineteenth century, was that symptomatic hemorrhoids were due to vascular hyperplasia. The anal submucosa was thought to be erectile and piles resulted from hyperplasia of the "corpus cavernosum recti." The bright red nature of the bleeding was then explained by the existence of arteriovenous communications.

The third theory from the 1950s was that hemorrhoids resulted from degeneration of supportive tissue in the anal canal, and this concept is corroborated by more recent studies. In 1975 Thomson published a summary of his thesis during in which he studied 95 cadaveric anorectal specimens in combination with a clinical study of 80 patients admitted for treatment of piles [1]. He was the first to describe cushions of submucosal tissue in the anal canal present in asymptomatic patients. These "anal cushions" were present in a triradiate appearance (left lateral, right anterior, and right posterior; or more commonly at 3, 7, and 11 o'clock) and composed of blood vessels, Treiz's muscle, and elastic and connective tissue. These structures are identifiable in early embryonic life.

D. Jayne and A. Stuto (eds.), *Transanal Stapling Techniques for Anorectal Prolapse,*
DOI: 10.1007/978-1-84800-905-9_3, © Springer-Verlag London Limited 2009

The anal cushions are essential for continence and act as an anal plug at rest. The internal sphincter, as a muscle cylinder, cannot close the anal canal completely, but requires a distensible lining (the anal cushions) to produce a water-tight seal. The vascular spaces of the anal cushions are supplied directly from the arterial system, and at low sphincter pressures they are thought to swell whereas at higher pressures they become compressed, effectively maintaining continence at the extremes of anal pressure. Indeed, the vascular filling probably accounts for 15–20% of resting anal canal pressure. These theories may explain why Milligan–Morgan hemorrhoidectomy with excision of the anal cushions sometimes results in seepage and passive incontinence.

Thomson's work showed that the pathology of resected piles showed no relationship with vascular hyperplasia as previously suspected, but that a rich network of dilated capillaries existed in the lamina propria. Symptomatic bleeding was associated with dilatation of these capillaries. Further work by Haas and Fox found that the mucosa and the skin of the anal canal are anchored by connective tissue fibers to the internal sphincter and to a connective tissue mesh between the muscle fibers of the sphincter [5]. This mesh is then anchored to the conjoined longitudinal coat of the anal canal. With age connective tissue fibers deteriorate and fail to anchor the mucosa and the anal cushions to the internal sphincter. This results in the cushions being forced down by vertical forces during straining with bulging out through the anus.

The current theory is therefore that piles are caused by a sliding anal lining with prolapse resulting when Trietz's muscle is repeatedly stretched along with degeneration and fragmentation of the supporting connective tissue.

Classification of Hemorrhoids

The term hemorrhoids is generally used to describe enlarged anal cushions which become symptomatic through bleeding or prolapse. However, correlation between symptoms and hemorrhoidal appearance is poor. In a series of 835 patients, hemorrhoids were seen on examination in 82% of asymptomatic and 88% of symptomatic patients [6]. It should be kept in mind that prolapsed hemorrhoids may be asymptomatic, particularly in the elderly female with low anal pressure, whereas normal-looking anal cushions may cause severe symptoms, most notably in males with high anal tone.

The most widely used classification of hemorrhoids is that attributed to Goligher, which describes four grades/degrees based on the clinical appearance (Table 3.1 and Fig. 3.1). Although this system has its strengths in that it is symptom based and easy to apply, it does have its limitations. It fails to take into consideration any symptoms other than bleeding and prolapse and ignores the fact that bleeding may not be due to piles. There is also the tendency for clinicians to overstage hemorrhoids based on clinical appearance rather than patient-reported prolapse. Patients are frequently confused about the symptoms of prolapse, describing it in vague terms as a "lump" or "something coming down" during the act of defecation. Such a "lump" might easily be confused with external hemorrhoids or skin tags rather than true internal hemorrhoidal prolapse.

The need for a more refined classification of hemorrhoidal disease has long been recognized, particularly with the increasing therapeutic options available and the need to compare outcomes of clinical trials. To this end, Nicholls and Glass [7] described a 4-stage classification system with an emphasis on treatment choice:

1. *Occasional symptoms*: reassurance after exclusion of colorectal disease is all that is required
2. *Bleeding with no prolapse*: treatment with suppositories or injection is likely to be helpful
3. *Prolapse*: rubber band ligation may be indicated
4. *Prolapse with large symptomatic external component*: conservative measures are unlikely to help, and hemorrhoidectomy is the treatment of choice

This classification, although clinically useful, is now somewhat outdated by the increasing array of therapeutic interventions available for symptomatic piles.

TABLE 3.1. Goligher's classification of hemorrhoids.

Grade	Symptoms
I	Bleed but do not prolapse
II	Prolapse during defecation but reduce spontaneously
III	Prolapse and require manual reduction
IV	Permanently prolapse and cannot be reduced

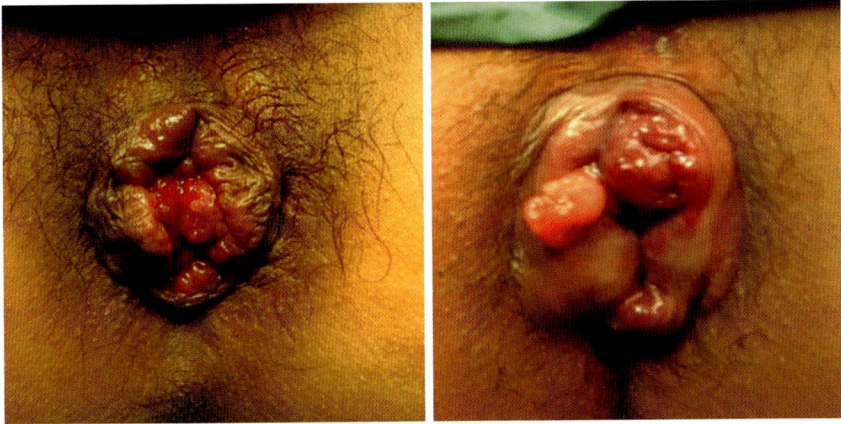

FIG. 3.1. Degrees of hemorrhoidal prolapse. (a) Third-degree prolapse becomes apparent on straining and requires manual reduction, (b) fourth-degree permanently prolapsed hemorrhoids

TABLE 3.2. Classification of hemorrhoids as proposed by Lunnis [10].

Stage	Morphology	Presentation	Additional features	Size
Nonprolapsing				
0	Anal cushions	Bleed very rarely No prolapse	None	No definite increase
1	Small hemorrhoids	Bleed intermittently No prolapse	None	Minor definite increase
Prolapsing				
2	Intermediate hemorrhoids	Prolapse but return spontaneously Bleed frequently and sometimes profusely	Pruritis Skin tags rare	Moderate increased size which prolapse on straining
3	Large hemorrhoids	Prolapse and need aid to reduce	Pruritis Discomfort	Major increase in size, including circumferential
		Bleed frequently and often profusely	Some skin tags common	Prolapse easily and require replacement
4	Very large ± additional features	Prolapse which is permanent and irreducible	Pain	Extreme increase in size
		Bleed profusely which can soil underwear	Pruritis, soiling Many skin tags usual Bleed profusely which can soil underwear Complications, e.g., thrombosis	Secondary hemorrhoids Skin tags

Recent attempts to produce a more accurate and reliable classification of symptomatic hemorrhoids have included the work of the Gaj [8, 9] and Lunniss [10]. In the discussion paper from Lunniss, the requirements for an ideal classification for hemorrhoids are presented along with a proposed system (Table 3.2). Further attempts at classifying hemorrhoidal disease have included the use of flexible endoscopic evaluation rather than traditional rigid protoscopy. Using these techniques attempts have been made to correlate the endoscopic appearance of hemorrhoids with their symptomatology [11] and the results of therapeutic intervention [12]. Although the endoscopic appearance of hemorrhoids does appear to be predictive of response to local treatments, the technique has not been fully evaluated in relation to excisional hemorrhoidectomy.

Hemorrhoidal Symptoms

Hemorrhoidal symptoms may mimic a multitude of other anal and rectal conditions. Indeed, patients and nonmedical personnel frequently attribute most anal symptom to piles, which results in estimates of prevalence as high as 86% [6].

Hemorrhoidal symptoms may include one or more of the following complaints to varying degrees: bleeding, anal swelling and prolapse, discomfort or pain, anal discharge and pruritis, and anal hygiene and cosmesis. In general terms, the larger the degree of prolapse, the more symptomatic the hemorrhoids.

Bleeding

This is the most common hemorrhoidal complaint. It is typically bright red and may be distinguished from the similar fresh bleeding of an anal fissure by the lack of accompanying anal pain. In the early stages, the bleeding is noticed on the toilet paper, separate from the stool. As the degree of prolapse progresses, the bleeding becomes more profuse, dripping into the toilet pan or splattering the pan at the end of defecation. This typically occurs when the congested anal cushions prolapse beyond the anal sphincter. In the most advanced stages, when the mucosal prolapse is permanently outside the anus, there may be a bright red bloody mucous discharge unrelated to defecation. It is unusual for bleeding to be severe enough to cause anemia, although this has been reported to occur in 0.5 patients per 100,000 population [13]. This may be more common in patients with portal hypertension.

Prolapse and Lump

Prolapse is experienced by the patients as a sensation of "something coming down" or a "lump" at the anal verge that may require manual digitation to reduce it. However, it can often be difficult to elicit a concise history of prolapse, and verification by examination is always required. Patients can readily confuse a lump at the anal verge as hemorrhoidal prolapse, when in fact it may be due to an edematous anal skin tag, a thrombosed perianal vein, or a hypertrophied anal papilla (fibroepithelial polyp).

Mucous Discharge, Pruritis, and Hygiene Difficulties

Persistent hemorrhoidal prolapse at the anal verge causes irritation of the mucous membrane covering the hemorrhoidal tissue, giving rise to mucous discharge with or without blood staining that soils the underwear. This can cause symptoms of "wetness" leading to pruritis with irritation and itching of the perianal skin.

Anal skin tags are thought to represent "gravestones to hemorrhoids past" but may in fact develop de novo. They may present with problems in perianal hygiene, causing pruritis and soiling, or for reasons of cosmesis.

Pain and Discomfort

Uncomplicated hemorrhoidal disease is usually painless. However, patients will frequently describe a discomfort or a dull ache in the anus after defecation. This may be relieved by reduction of the prolapse. Presentation with severe anal pain should therefore prompt a search for an alternative diagnosis, such as an anal fissure, carcinoma, or perianal sepsis. However, the coexistence of hemorrhoidal prolapse and anal fissures is not uncommon, particularly in those patients with high anal canal pressures. Pain may also be a feature of hemorrhoidal thrombosis, but this will be obvious on clinical examination.

Constipation is often reported by patients suffering from piles, but most have a normal bowel frequency and some actually have disorders associated with a diarrheal state [14]. It is more probable that the hemorrhoids cause a sense of constipation or that the history of constipation follows the piles rather than predates it. Certainly, one must be wary of the diagnosis of solitary hemorrhoidal prolapse when symptoms of obstructed defecation exist. In such circumstances, the hemorrhoidal prolapse is likely to be just part of a more significant anorectal prolapse that requires further investigation.

Cultural, educational, and socioeconomic factors will influence the presentation of patients with piles and the acceptance of the clinical symptoms resulting from bleeding or prolapsing anal cushions. Indeed several studies have shown that people in the higher socioeconomic groups more frequently report hemorrhoids. A positive family history is common, which may be cultural, dietary, behavioral, or genetic.

Hemorrhoids: Differential Diagnosis

It is obviously important to exclude a diagnosis of neoplasia in any patient presenting with rectal bleeding. For this reason, most authorities would recommend a flexible sigmoidoscopic evaluation in all patients over the age of 40 years. Most other diseases of the anorectum can be diagnosed with a combination of visual and digital examination of the anorectum, supplemented by proctoscopy and rigid sigmoidoscopy. A list of differential diagnoses to consider when investigating hemorrhoidal disease is given in Table 3.3. One should keep in mind that it is possible for symptomatic hemorrhoids to coexist with all these conditions.

Clinical Assessment

Patients presenting with symptoms of hemorrhoids should have a thorough examination in order to exclude alternative or coexisting pathologies of the anorectum.

Inspection

Inspection of the perianal region is best performed with the patient lying comfortably in the left lateral (Sims) position with adequate lighting. The presence of anal skin tags is an obvious sign of previous hemorrhoidal prolapse. There may be maceration or a dermatitis of the perianal skin if seepage and pruritis is a feature. Evidence of previous obstetric trauma (episiotomy or sutured tear) should be looked for as an indication of compromised anal canal pressure. Large fourth-degree hemorrhoids will be obvious as they prolapse through the anal verge, but third-degree piles may require gentle eversion of the anal margin to become evident. If the patient can be persuaded to bear down, second-degree piles may be seen transiently descending into the anal canal. Eversion of the anus will also enable the majority of fissures to be detected.

Palpation

Digital rectal examination is of limited value in the assessment of hemorrhoidal prolapse. Hemorrhoids by virtue of their blood filled content are soft and compressible and cannot be quantified by the examining finger. A crude assessment of anal canal pressure, both at rest and on squeeze, is possible and may provide some guidance in the choice of therapeutic intervention. If present, the finding of a weak sphincter should be confirmed with the use of physiology and ultrasound evaluation. Digital rectal examination in patients with hemorrhoidal disease is usually not associated with pain, unless there is hemorrhoidal thrombosis. The finding of pain suggests a possible fissure, perianal sepsis, or anorectal cancer.

Proctoscopy

Proctoscopy is the mainstay in the diagnosis of hemorrhoids. A well-lubricated, lighted proctoscope is gently inserted fully into the distal rectum. This has the effect of reducing the internal piles. The obturator is then removed and the proctoscope slowly retracted. As the proctoscope is withdrawn any prolapsing piles will be visible bulging into the proctoscope lumen, and their size and location should be recorded. Although a straight proctoscope is frequently used in the assessment of hemorrhoids, the extent of any prolapse is probably best appreciated with a beveled proctoscope. Such an instrument has to be reinserted several times to observe the whole anorectal circumference. The enhanced view greatly facilitates the application of local treatments (Fig. 3.2).

TABLE 3.3. Differential diagnosis in hemorrhoidal disease.

Symptoms	Differential diagnosis
Pain	Fissure
	Abscess/fistula
Bleeding	Fissure
	Colorectal polyp
	Colorectal cancer
	Proctitis
Discharge/pruritis	Hypertrophic anal papilla
	Fistula
	Condylomata (anal warts)
	Rectal prolapse
	Anal incontinence
Lump or prolapse	Hypertrophic anal papilla
	Abscess
	Anal skin tag
	Perianal Crohn's disease

A   B

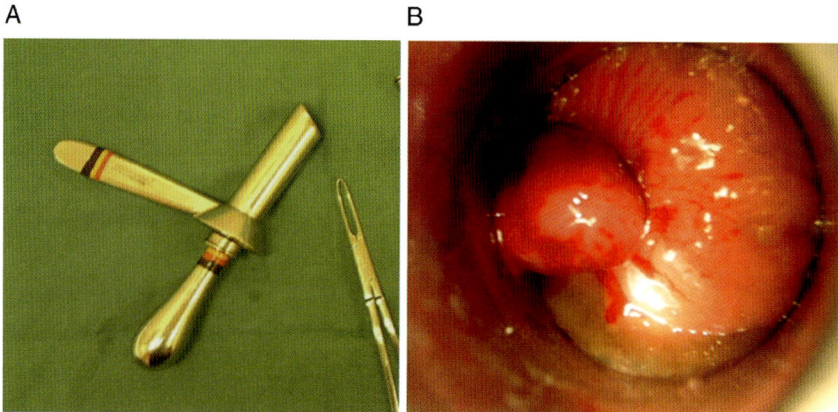

F<small>IG.</small> 3.2. (a) The beveled proctoscope facilitates viewing of hemorrhoidal prolapse, (b) view down the beveled proctoscope following application of a rubber band

Sigmoidoscopy and Colonoscopy

It cannot be stated too frequently that just because hemorrhoids are present they are not necessarily the source of fresh rectal bleeding. Any history of fresh bleeding in a patient over 40 years of age requires further investigation by means of flexible sigmoidoscopy to exclude colorectal neoplasia. If the patient is under 40 years of age, and the history is very much that of anal canal bleeding, then it is probably sufficient to limit endoscopic evaluation to a rigid sigmoidoscopy. This will exclude the majority of rectal pathologies including proctitis. The caveat is that further colonic investigation will be necessary if the bleeding does not respond to therapeutic measures. If there is any doubt about the diagnosis, or if there is a family history of colorectal neoplasia, then the rest of the colon will need investigation preferably by colonoscopy.

Anorectal Physiology and Endoanal Ultrasound

Anorectal physiology and endoanal ultrasound have a limited place in the routine evaluation of hemorrhoidal disease. They are occasionally of value in evaluating coexistent anal sphincter injury, but seldom have an impact on management. Excessive surgical removal of hemorrhoidal tissue in patients with low anal pressures may predispose them to seepage and soiling. The majority of patients with symptomatic hemorrhoids, however, will have elevated anal pressure, usually secondary to raised internal sphincter tone. Those patients with excessively elevated pressures will have a tendency to severe pain following excisional surgery.

Having completed the process of inspection, palpation, and examination, the clinician should have excluded most other anorectal pathologies and be in a position to classify the extent of hemorrhoidal disease. The extent of disease then needs to be correlated with the assessment of symptoms gained from the history. On the basis of this a management plan can be formulated.

The Diagnosis of Hemorrhoidal Complications

Internal Hemorrhoidal Thrombosis

Thrombosis of the internal hemorrhoids usually occurs in patients with a previous history of reducible hemorrhoidal prolapse, but may occur as the first manifestation of disease. It is associated with intense pain that limits sitting, walking, or defecation. The thrombosed, prolapsed piles are readily visible at the anal margin as a congested, tender mass surrounded by edematous perianal skin (Fig. 3.3). The thrombosed pile may be solitary or may involve several pedicles in which circumstance there may be diagnostic confusion with a small full-thickness rectal prolapse. If left untreated there is the potential for hemorrhoidal infarction, which should be suspected if there is accompanying pyrexia or systemic illness. In such circumstances,

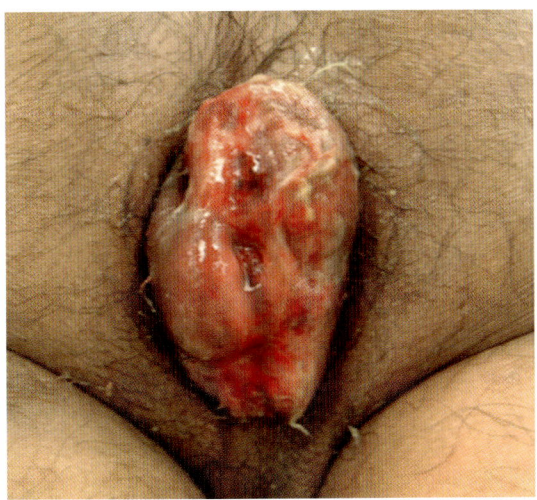

Fig. 3.3. Acute hemorrhoidal prolapse with thrombosis

urgent examination under anesthesia and limited hemorrhoidectomy should be performed.

Anemia

Hemorrhoidal bleeding is a rare cause of anemia. However, it is occasionally seen and is probably more common in premenopausal women, patients with portal hypertension, and those with blood dyscrasias or on anticoagulant therapy. The important point to note is that if anemia is present, then another source of bleeding, such as a peptic ulcer or a colorectal neoplasm, should always be considered.

Perianal Hematoma

The commonly used term "perianal hematoma" actually refers to intravascular thrombosis of the external anal veins [15]. It is not actually part of the spectrum of internal hemorrhoidal disease as it presents as a separate unrelated swelling on the anal verge which does not communicate with the anal canal. It is readily diagnosed by gentle parting of the buttocks which reveals a smooth, tense, bluish swelling which is exquisitively tender to touch.

Perianal Dermatitis

Perianal dermatitis occurs as a result of maceration due to mucous discharge from permanently prolapsed piles, as a consequence of poor anal hygiene associated with skin tags, or as a result of a local sensitivity reaction to topical drugs. The principles of management include attention to anal hygiene and the avoidance of moisturizing agents which will exacerbate skin maceration. In exceptional circumstances where pruritis and itching is a predominant symptom, a short course of topical antihistamine may be beneficial to break the cycle of pruritis, scratching, and further skin trauma.

Obstructed Defecation Syndrome

Definition of Obstructed Defecation Syndrome

Obstructed defecation syndrome is best defined as the normal desire to defecate but an inability to satisfactorily evacuate the rectum. It falls under the more general term "constipation." Most clinicians use the word constipation to refer to infrequent, incomplete, difficult, or prolonged evacuation or to describe the difficult passage of hard stools. The term constipation is therefore all encompassing and fails to discriminate colonic from rectal causes of defecatory dysfunction. It portrays little information about the underlying etiology or the potential treatment options. It is far better to divide patients with constipation into those with slow-transit constipation (colonic inertia) and those with obstructed defecation (pelvic outlet obstruction), accepting that there will be a population that displays a mixed picture. This terminology has a direct relevance to investigation and treatment.

Symptoms of Obstructed Defecation Syndrome

As with any syndrome, obstructed defecation encompasses a multitude of symptoms and may include one or more of the following:

1. Prolonged straining to open the bowels
2. Excessive time spent on the toilet to achieve evacuation
3. A sensation of incomplete evacuation
4. Frequent visits to the toilet to empty the rectum and the passage of small quantities of stool-fragmented defecation
5. A dependence on laxatives or enemas to achieve evacuation

6. The need for manual assistance to initiate evacuation
7. Anorectal discomfort or pain
8. Fresh rectal bleeding
9. A sensation of anorectal prolapse

There is a general reluctance to discuss rectal function and habit, and as a consequence many patients do not seek medical advice, preferring to self-treat using over-the-counter medications. Because of this there is a tendency for only the more severe end of the spectrum to present to the coloproctologist: the so-called iceberg phenomenon. By the time the patient is seen in the outpatient clinic, the condition has often been going on for several years. There is a tendency for the patient's daily routine to be dictated by their bowel function and their behavior to appear obsessive. In the past this has led to the erroneous labelling of many of these patients as suffering from psychological problems. Similarly, allegations of previous sexual abuse in these patients have not been substantiated. It is likely that these inappropriate labels have arisen from the ignorance of the medical fraternity, based on a limited understanding of the underlying pathophysiology. Although some psychiatric and psychological disorders do manifest as rectal evacuatory dysfunction, this should not be assumed until appropriate investigations have excluded an organic cause.

The typical patient with obstructed defecation is the multiparous female, although it is observed in some 5% of males and occasionally in young nulliparous females. Many have undergone previous pelvic surgery, most usually hysterectomy, gynecological prolapse repair, or surgery for anorectal conditions, such hemorrhoids. As described earlier, there may be some overlap with symptoms of slow-transit constipation or coexistent irritable bowel syndrome.

A careful history can go a long way to discriminating slow-transit constipation from obstructed defecation. Thus, patients with slow-transit constipation frequently describe infrequent bowel motions, but between bowel movements there is no desire to defecate. This contrasts to the constant desire to defecate described by patients with obstructed defecation. The lack of bowel movements in patients with slow-transit constipation is frequently accompanied by abdominal bloating or pain, which is eased by the passage of a formed or a hard motion. Abdominal bloating or pain is less frequently seen in isolated obstructed defecation, unless there are coexistent irritable bowel symptoms, and the motions are usually normally formed and soft.

The typical patient with obstructed defecation will describe a long history of defecatory complaints which are usually progressive over the course of several years. Occasionally, a precipitating event, such as a previous hysterectomy, will be described. Although it is more common in multiparous females, there does not appear to be any definite relation to the number of pregnancies or births. The patient has a normal or a heightened appreciation of the need to defecate. This prompts a visit to the toilet where, despite repeated straining efforts, rectal emptying is either unsuccessful or occurs as the passage of small, fragmented pieces of motion. The patient may be aware of a bulging of the stool (rectum) into the vagina, characteristic of a rectocele. Alternatively, the patient may refer to the stool "going the wrong way" or to a "blockage" being present. In order to redirect the stool or overcome the blockage, the patient may find inserting a finger into the vagina or rectum, or supporting the perineum in some other way, as being beneficial in initiating defecation. The end result is that the patient is left with a feeling of incomplete rectal evacuation, which in turn prompts a return to the toilet sometime later and so the cycle repeats itself. Laxatives and enemas are frequently helpful, and the patient becomes dependent on them to achieve evacuation. Repeated straining exacerbates the problem, promoting anorectal prolapse which may cause bleeding and discomfort or rarely pain.

It should be appreciated that obstructed defecation is often a manifestation of a more global pelvic floor problem, with some 30–40% of patients having symptoms of a urogynecological nature. For this reason, it is recommended that all patients with obstructed defecation are best assessed in a combined pelvic floor clinic, with input from a gynecologist, a nurse specialist, and a physiotherapist with an interest in pelvic floor dysfunction. This will streamline investigations and facilitate combined operative interventions if necessary.

When treating patients with obstructed defecation it should be kept in mind that it is a benign condition, and as such the outcome of treatment is to improve quality of life. The use of a standardized interview questionnaire, encompassing all aspects of pelvic floor function, is to be encouraged as is the use of a quality-of-life instrument. Several quality-of-life tools exist. These may assess the impact of bowel function alone on quality of life [16], or better still may assess pelvic floor function in its entirety [17].

Several attempts have been made to quantitate obstructed defecation symptoms with the use of scoring systems. This is particularly useful for comparing symptoms before and after treatment or when analyzing clinical trials. The most commonly referred to scoring system in terms of obstructed defecation, and with particular reference to the STARR procedure, is Longo's ODS score (Table 3.4). Although this has been used in most studies of STARR for obstructed defecation it has never been formally validated and suffers from several inherent weaknesses (see Chap. 9). Recent attempts to improve on Longo's ODS score include those by Altomare [18], Varma [19], and Knowles [20]. In particular those scoring systems proposed by Varma and Knowles incorporate an analysis of obstructed defecation symptoms in an attempt to distinguish it from slow-transit constipation.

Clinical Assessment

When a history suggestive of obstructed defecation has been obtained, the clinician should focus his examination not only on rectal anatomy and function but also on other pathologies associated with pelvic floor prolapse. Again, combined input with examination by a coloproctologist as well as a urogynecologist is beneficial. Abnormalities of the pelvic organs detectable on clinical examination may include anterior rectocele, rectal intussusception, enterocele, vaginal or uterine prolapse, and cystocele. However, for the purposes of this chapter attention will be focused on the clinical findings of the posterior pelvic compartment (anorectum).

If the patient is to undergo combined examination by a urogynecologist and a coloproctologist, it is usual for the gynecologist to perform vaginal examination first with the patient lying in the supine position with the hips and knees flexed.

TABLE 3.4. Longo's original obstructed defecation syndrome (ODS) scoring system.

Frequency of defecation	Score
1–2 defecations every 1–2 days	0
2 Defecations/week or 3 defecations or attempts/day	1
1 Defecation/week or 4 defecations or attempts/day	2
<1 Defecation/week or >4 defecations or attempts/day	3
Intensity of straining	
No or light	0
Moderate	1
Intense	2
Duration of straining	
Short	1
Prolonged or many times	2
Incomplete evacuation	
Never	0
≤1×/week	1
2×/week	2
>2×/week	3
Rectoperineal discomfort	
Never	0
≤1×/week	1
2×/week	2
>2×/week	3
Reduction of activities	
None	0
<25% of activity	2
25–50% of activity	4
>50% of activity	6
Laxatives	
Never	0
<25% of defecations	1
25–50% of defecations	3
>50% of defecations	5
Always	7
Enemas	
Never	0
<25% of defecations	1
25–50% of defecations	3
>50% of defecations	5
Always	7
Digitation	
Never	0
<25% of defecations	1
25–50% of defecations	3
>50% of defecations	5
Always	7

Once this is complete, the patient turns into the left lateral (Sims) position.

Inspection of the perianal region may reveal a patulous anus if there is accompanying sphincter weakness, or skin tags if there are coexistent hemorrhoids. It is useful to ask the patient to strain down, and for this purpose a piece of tissue paper is held against the anus and the patient reassured that he/she will not make a mess. Straining allows a rough estimation to be made about the degree of perineal descent or laxity of the pelvic floor. It will also enable any mucohemorrhoidal prolapse or full-thickness rectal prolapse to be observed.

Digital rectal examination allows an impression to be formed regarding the resting and squeeze pressures generated by the anal sphincter, and any obvious sphincter defects or deficiencies of the perineal body can be palpated. Anteriorly, the lower rectovaginal septum is palpated for the presence of a rectocele with its typical bulging into the vagina.

Proctoscopic examination is useful in determining any associated hemorrhoidal prolapse. In addition, the proctoscope can be withdrawn to the level of the anorectal ring and the patient asked to strain; any internal rectal prolapse (intussusception) may be visible prolapsing into the open end of the proctoscope. Bearing down also gives an impression of the patient's ability to expel the proctoscope from the distal rectum and anus. Proctoscopy is complemented by rigid sigmoidoscopy, which eliminates coexistent rectal cancer, inflammatory bowel disease, and solitary rectal ulcer. Rarely, gross internal rectal prolapse may be evident on flexible sigmoidoscopy (Fig. 3.4), which is performed mainly to exclude coexistent colorectal disease.

Having taken a careful history and thorough examination, the clinician should be in a position to reach a preliminary diagnosis upon which to base subsequent investigation. Specifically, it should be possible to discriminate to some degree whether the patient is suffering from slow-transit constipation,

obstructed defecation, or a mixture of the two. It should also be possible to determine whether rectal evacuatory dysfunction exists in isolation or is in combination with other pelvic floor prolapse. Confirmation of the clinical assessment will require further investigation, which is described elsewhere (Chap. 4).

References

1. Thomson WHF. The nature of haemorrhoids. Br J Surg 1975; 62: 542–552
2. Parks AG. De haemorrhois. Guy's Hosp Rep 1955; 104: 135
3. Morgagni JG. Seats and causes of disease. Letter 32 Article 10 Translated by Benjamin Alexander. 1769; 2: 105 London: Millar
4. Allingham W, Allingham HW. The diagnosis and treatment of diseases of the rectum. 7th edn, London: Bailliere, 1901
5. Haas PA, Fox TA. Age-related changes and scar formations of perianal connective tissue. Dis Colon Rectum 1980; 23: 160–169
6. Haas PA, Fox TA, Haas GP. The pathogenesis of haemorrhoids. Dis Colon Rectum 1984; 27: 442–450
7. Nicholls RJ, Glass RE. Coloproctology: diagnosis and outpatient management. Berlin: Springer, 1985
8. Gaj F, Trecca A. PATE 2000 Sorrento: a modern, effective instrument for defining haemorrhoids. A multicentre observational study conducted in 930 symptomatic patients. Chir Ital 2004; 56: 509–515
9. Gaj F, Trecca A. New "PATE 2006" system for classifying haemorrhoidal disease: advantages resulting from revision of "PATE 2000 Sorrento". Chir Ital 2007; 59: 521–526
10. Lunniss PJ, Mann CV. Classification of internal haemorrhoids: a discussion paper. Colorectal Dis 2004; 6: 226–232
11. Sadahiro S, Mukai M, Tokunaga N, Tajima T, Makuuchi H. A new method of evaluating hemorrhoids with the retroflexed fiberoptic colonoscope. Gastrointest Endosc 1998; 48: 272–275
12. Fukuda A, Kajiyama T, Kishimoto H, Arakawa H, Someda H, Sakai M, Seno H, Chiba T. Colonoscopic classification of internal hemorrhoids: usefulness in endoscopic band ligation. J Gastroenterol Hepatol 2005; 20: 46–50
13. Kluiber RM, Wolf BG. Evaluation of anaemia caused by hemorrhoidal bleeding. Dis Colon Rectum 1994; 37: 1006–1007
14. Delco F, Sonnenberg A. Associations between hemorrhoids and other diagnoses. Dis Colon Rectum 1998; 41: 1534–1541

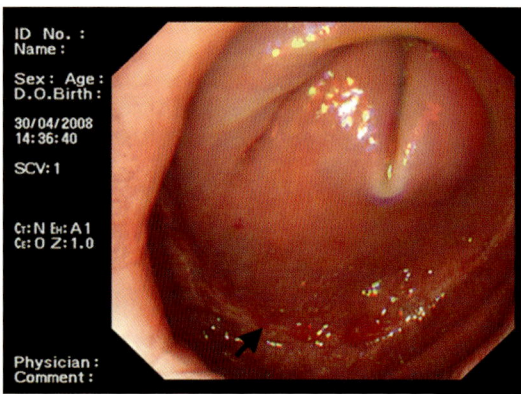

FIG. 3.4. Internal rectal prolapse as observed through a flexible sigmoidoscope. A previous stapled hemorrhoidopexy line can be seen (*arrowhead*), which has failed to treat the symptomatic prolapse

15. Thomson WHF. The nature of perianal haematoma. Lancet 1982; ii: 467

16. Marquist P, De La Loge C, Dubois D, McDermott A, Chassaney O. Development and validation of the patient assessment of constipation quality of life questionnaire. Scand J Gastroenterol 2005; 40: 540–551

17. e-PAQ: Electronic Patient Assessment. http://www.epaq.co.uk

18. Altomare DF, Spazzafuma L, Rinaldi M, Dodi G, Ghiselli R, Piloni V. Set-up and statistical validation of a new scoring system for obstructed defaecation syndrome. Colorectal Dis 2008; 10: 84–88

19. Varma MG, Wang JY, Berian JR, Patterson BA, McCrea GL, Hart SL. The constipation severity instrument: a validated measure. Dis Colon Rectum 2008; 51: 162–172

20. Knowles CH, Eccersley AJ, Scott SM, Walker SM, Reeves B, Lunniss PJ. Linear discriminant analysis of symptoms in patients with chronic constipation: validation of a new scoring system (KESS). Dis Colon Rectum 2000; 43: 1419–1426

Chapter 4
Evaluation of Patients with Symptomatic Hemorrhoids and Obstructed Defecation

F. Pigot, F.H. Hetzer, and J.-J. Tuech

Abstract The diagnosis of both hemorrhoids and obstructed defecation syndrome (ODS) starts with a careful history and clinical examination. Thus it is supplemented, where necessary, with specific investigations aimed at characterizing the nature of the underlying pathophysiology and defining coexistent disease. This chapter describes the various investigations that are available to the coloproctologist in the investigations of hemorrhoids and ODS, their indications, and their relative usefulness in influencing clinical management.

Introduction

For the vast majority of patients suffering from hemorrhoidal symptoms, laboratory evaluation may be minimal. The basic work-up has three aims. Firstly, to confirm hemorrhoidal disease, as symptoms may be nonspecific and symptomatic hemorrhoids may have a grossly normal appearance. Secondly, to assess anorectal anatomy and physiology and to exclude coexistent pathology that might modify the surgical approach. Thirdly, to assess patients after hemorrhoidal surgery where there has been an alteration of anorectal function, leading to new symptoms.

Investigation of Hemorrhoidal Disease

As with any other medical condition, the evaluation of hemorrhoidal symptoms begins with a careful and thorough history and clinical examination. This will reveal most of the information that the clinician requires to formulate a management plan. Further investigation aims to confirm the diagnosis, document its severity, and exclude the presence of coexistent pathology. We describe the investigations that might be considered as a supplement to history and clinical examination.

Rigid Sigmoidoscopy and Proctoscopy

Rigid sigmoidoscopy and proctoscopy should be performed on every patient presenting with hemorrhoidal symptoms. These examinations are easy to perform and well tolerated in the outpatient setting. They should be combined with a digital rectal examination to assess sphincter integrity and squeeze ability and to determine any coexistent rectocele. Rigid sigmoidoscopy in the unprepared patient can usually provide sufficient views of most of the rectum, but complete examination may require the use of an enema preparation. It is a cheap and effective means of eliminating proctitis, polyps, or tumors. Proctoscopy confirms the presence of enlarged hemorrhoids and helps to corroborate the degree of prolapse in terms of patient report symptoms. Asking the patient to push down, as if attempting to open his/her bowels, with the proctoscope inserted gives an indication of any coexistent internal rectal prolapse.

Flexible Sigmoidoscopy and Colonoscopy

Hemorrhoidal symptoms can to be nonspecific, comprising one of more of rectal bleeding,

D. Jayne and A. Stuto (eds.), *Transanal Stapling Techniques for Anorectal Prolapse*,
DOI: 10.1007/978-1-84800-905-9_4, © Springer-Verlag London Limited 2009

anorectal discomfort, prolapse, mucous discharge, and pruritis. These symptoms are shared with a variety of other colorectal pathologies (inflammatory, neoplasia, infectious, etc). The clinical dilemma is in selecting those patients whose symptoms warrant further investigation without subjecting everyone to the rigors of colonoscopic examination. It can be further debated whether selected patients should undergo full colonoscopy or whether flexible sigmoidoscopic examination of the left colon alone is sufficient.

As most inflammatory and infective conditions will be apparent at rigid sigmoidoscopy, the main aim of flexible endoscopic examination to exclude the presence of neoplasia (polyps and cancers). Full colonoscopic evaluation is recommended in all patients with a family history of colorectal neoplasia or when hemorrhoidal symptoms are combined with other "red-flag" symptoms, including a recent history of altered bowel habit, weight loss, abdominal pain, and anemia. Given the natural history of colorectal neoplasia, the threshold for colonoscopic evaluation should probably be reduced in those over the age of 50 years.

In patients presenting with isolated anal canal-type bleeding, typified by the painless passage of fresh blood during or after defecation, it is probably sufficient to restrict examination to flexible sigmoidoscopy. Whether rigid sigmoidoscopy alone is sufficient in younger patients, less than 40 years, is debatable. On the one hand it is stated that some 20% of endoscopic examinations will be abnormal in this age group of patients presenting with rectal bleeding, with polyps being the most frequent abnormality. However, other series have reported no cancers and only a 4% polyp detection rate when flexible sigmoidoscopy was performed in patients less than 55 years with isolated fresh rectal bleeding and a clinically apparent cause, such as hemorrhoids or anal fissure [1]. Similarly, when the diagnosis of cancer was made at colonoscopy, in 80% etiology other than hemorrhoids was clinically suspected [2]. Thus, it would appear that in younger patients, of 40 years or less, it is probably sufficient to perform rigid sigmoidoscopic assessment of the rectum, provided the symptoms are of typical anal canal bleeding and in the absence of a family history of colorectal neoplasia or any other "red-flag" symptoms.

Anorectal Physiology

Anorectal physiology is rarely indicated in patients with uncomplicated hemorrhoidal disease, but should be reserved for those patients with symptoms of incontinence, obstructed defecation, or suspected occult obstetric sphincter injury. For this reason, all patients presenting with hemorrhoidal symptoms should specifically be questioned about the existence of incontinence, obstructed defecation, and past obstetric experience. Sphincter dysfunction revealed preoperatively may alter the decision to perform excisional surgery, and if surgery is to be performed which intervention is preferred.

Resting anal canal pressures are characteristically higher in patients with hemorrhoidal disease than normal controls. Anal hypertonia may be due to internal sphincter hyperactivity, with a high frequency (30–50%) of ultraslow waves being present [3]. Alternatively, the increased resting pressure may be attributed to the presence of engorged hemorrhoidal cushions within the anal canal, which would explain the relatively normal resting pressures observed in individuals with prolapsing hemorroidal disease [4]. Anal squeeze pressures do not differ significantly from normal controls.

Excessive straining at defecation is frequently observed in patients with hemorrhoidal disease and may be associated with perineal descent and pudendal neuropathy [5]. However, the manometric profile is not altered to the same extent as in patients with obstructed defecation and descending perineum syndrome [6].

Rectal sensation to balloon inflation is usually normal and the rectoanal inhibitory reflex preserved. However, a smaller reduction in anal canal pressure may be seen in response to balloon inflation in patients with anal hypertonia or perineal neuropathy.

After hemorrhoidectomy, anal resting pressures reduce to values similar to controls with accompanying diminution in ultraslow wave activity [7–9]. The decrease in resting pressure may be associated with a temporary impairment in sphincter function, as demonstrated by abnormal fluid continence testing in patients 3 months after hemorrhoidectomy [10]. Decrease in elevated resting pressures may also be observed following successful rubber band ligation or injection sclerotherapy [11, 12].

Endoanal Ultrasound

Endoanal ultrasound in patients with symptomatic hemorrhoids is no different from controls. After conventional hemorrhoidectomy, internal and even external sphincter defects have been described, which may be asymptomatic or associated with new onset incontinence [13, 14]. Because of the risk of postoperative incontinence, it is recommended that anorectal ultrasound should be combined with anorectal physiology in the assessment of all patients with suspected or documented anal sphincter dysfunction, including those with a history of obstetric sphincter injury or previous anorectal surgery.

Defecography

Contrast defecography is rarely indicated in patients with hemorrhoidal symptoms. However, it should be considered in those patients with associated obstructed defecation symptoms and in those with significant internal rectal or other pelvic organ prolapse [15]. If performed, it may reveal a resting perineal position lower than in controls, but normal descent during straining [16].

Electromyography

Electromyography is normal in patients with uncomplicated hemorrhoidal disease. In those patients with associated obstructed defecation, some degree of neuropathy may be demonstrated. This test is only indicated in patients with a clinically suspected neurological defect, most commonly associated with incontinence.

Investigation of Obstructed Defecation

Introduction

Although a careful history and clinical examination will yield useful information in patients with obstructed defecation symptoms, rarely is it sufficient to enable an accurate assessment of the disease process. Although symptoms of excessive straining to defecate, fragmented defecation, incomplete evacuation, and fecal urgency may suggest a rectal evacuatory disorder, further radiological and physiological information is required to classify the disease and how it relates to overall pelvic floor function. From a clinical perspective it is helpful to categorize patients presenting with constipation into one of four categories (a) obstructed defecation, (b) slow transit, (c) mixed, and (d) normal. No single radiological or physiological investigation is able to accurately achieve this, but rather a battery of investigations is usually required [17–19]. Later we discuss the range of investigations available to the coloproctologist faced with a patient complaining of obstructed defecation, their indications and relatively usefulness. However, before undertaking any of these tests it is obviously necessary to exclude other colorectal pathology (neoplasia, inflammatory bowel disease, infection, etc.) by means of endoscopic examination in the form of either flexible sigmoidoscopy or colonoscopy.

Anorectal Physiology

Anorectal physiology should be performed according to a standardized protocol, which may be specific of each institution. Intraluminal anal canal pressure is measured with the patient lying in the left lateral position, at rest, with voluntary sphincter contraction, and during a simulated defecatory effort. Rectal sensation is evaluated by progressive inflation of an intrarectal rubber balloon. First sensation, permanent desire to defecate, and maximal tolerable volume are recorded. Anal pressure varies according to the probe diameter, and rectal sensation according to the protocol used for balloon inflation, therefore normal values must be determined in each center. In women, anal resting and squeeze pressures decrease after 50 years of age. The anal canal pressure profile is observed during progressive inflation of the intrarectal balloon. Normally, at around 40ml of inflation the lower anal canal pressure increases concomitantly with a decrease in that observed in the upper anal canal as a consequence of the rectoanal inhibitory reflex (RAIR).

Usually, the resting and maximal squeeze pressures in patients suffering from ODS are similar to controls [20]. However, in those patients with a long history of straining, especially when perineal descent is present (either at rest or on straining), the squeeze increment, maximal pressure amplitude, and duration of voluntary contraction may be lower, similar to that found in incontinent women [21]. Rarely, resting anal hypertonia is found, associated with the presence of ultraslow waves, particularly in those patients with pelvic floor dyssynergia [22].

The threshold volume required to evoke a first sensation is frequently higher in patients with ODS when compared to controls. However, the inflation volumes required to elicit a desire to defecate or to induce a feeling of urgency may not be different. Intrarectal pressures during straining tend to be lower in patients with obstructed defecation, even when the rectum is filled with a 60-ml air-inflated balloon [23].

The presence of a physiological megarectum is defined as a maximal tolerated rectal inflation volume in excess of 330ml. This abnormally is never found in asymptomatic subjects. In patients suffering from dyschezia its significance is debatable; patients with or without a megarectum do not differ in terms of clinical symptoms (except for the need to digitate with megarectum), past history of hysterectomy, sex, age, defecographic and manometric data (except for rectal sensation). Interestingly, antidepressive therapy is found more frequently in the megarectum group (33% vs. 11%) [24].

The RAIR may be low or absent in patients with severe constipation. As the absence of an intact RAIR is pathognomonic for congenital (Hirschprung's disease) or acquired (Chagas' disease) aganglionosis, further evaluation is mandatory in patients presenting with chronic constipation symptoms. When aganglionosis of the myenteric and submucosal plexuses is suspected, full-thickness rectal biopsies must be performed at various levels above the anal canal, because a wide variation in the density of ganglion cells at the anorectal junction has been observed in healthy individuals.

Characteristic manometric profiles are associated with certain anorectal disorders. In patients with a rectocele, the urge to defecate and maximal tolerated volumes are higher (mean: 100ml vs. 244ml, respectively) than in patients with ODS without a rectocele (67ml vs. 182ml, respectively). Intra-anal intussusception and external rectal prolapse are associated with a shorter anal canal length (1.9 and 2.9cm, respectively), and a lower resting anal pressure (44mmHg and 60mmHg, respectively) [25].

Pancolonic manometry is rarely performed in routine practice. It is indicated in some patients when there is a suspicion of colonic inertia. When performed in patients with ODS, it has shown a failure of propagation of colonic pressure waves prior to defecation [26].

Plain Radiology

Plain radiology is seldom of use in the diagnosis or management of obstructed defecation. Historically, it was used in the diagnosis of megarectum with a mean rectal diameter of >12cm, as measured at the pelvic brim following contrast instillation, being considered diagnostic [27]. However, this finding is too nonspecific to be of practical value. It is mostly found in patients with colon inertia.

Colonic Transit Studies

Counting the passage of ingested radio-opaque markers on plain abdominal X-rays gives an estimate of total and segmental colonic transit time. In the simplified method, 20 radio-opaque markers are ingested at the same time on days 1–3. Abdominal X-rays are obtained on days 4 and 7. Additional films are taken on day 10 in those patients with markers still present on the day 7 examination. The markers are identified and counted on the X-ray films. Projection zones of the right colon, left colon, and rectosigmoid are defined by the vertical lumbar axis and lines from the fifth lumbar vertebra to the anterior superior iliac spines. Colonic transit time in each segment and through the entire colon is calculated by multiplying the total number of pellets in each section by a factor of 1.2. Transit time is considered abnormal when its value exceeds the mean +2 standard deviations; for the right colon this is > 24h, the left colon > 31h, the rectosigmoid > 33h, and total colonic transit > 67h [28, 29].

Colonic transit time is prolonged in 80% of patients suffering from constipation with a low stool frequency and/or dyschezia. Low stool frequency is more frequent when transit time exceeds normal values. There is no correlation between anorectal physiological variables and global or segmental colonic transit time [30].

A prolonged rectosigmoid segmental transit time is found in 10–20% of constipated patients, either isolated or associated with a prolonged left colon transit. Rectosigmoid inertia is not specifically associated with symptoms of ODS or the general finding of pelvic floor dysfunction. The clinical presentation of patients with ODS is similar regardless of whether they have rectosigmoid inertia, right colonic inertia, left colonic inertia, or normal transit time, with the exception of the need to digitate to effect evacuation in those with rectosigmoid inertia. However, the need to digitate to effect defecation is not specific for rectosigmoid inertia, as it is also more frequent in patients with right colonic inertia when compared with other groups [31]. Rectosigmoid inertia has a high sensitivity but a low specificity in discriminating pelvic floor dysfunction from slow transit constipation or normal transit constipation [32].

Dynamic Defecography

The role of defecography in the evaluation of constipation is largely concerned with the identification of occult prolapses [31]. Defecography is crucial to the diagnosis and therapeutic decision making for patients with ODS. Although a good correlation exists between clinical and defecographic detection of rectocele and internal rectal prolapse, defecography has the added value of providing information on the anatomy and function of other pelvic organs.

Four contrast defecography with opacification of the rectum, vagina, bladder, and small bowel is now the preferred methodology. The patient receives a barium meal 1–2h before the examination to visualize the small bowel. Contrast medium is instilled into the vagina, the bladder, and the rectum. The patient is seated and X-rays are taken at rest, during squeezing, and during straining to defecate, and repeated until maximal rectal evacuation is achieved. Rectal morphology and the associated movements of the organs and pelvic floor are recorded. The anorectal angle is measured as that between the axis of the anal canal and the median rectal axis (or posterior rectal wall tangential axis). Perineal position is defined as the position of the anorectal junction in relation to the inferior ischial plane or a line drawn from the pubic symphysis and the tip of the coccyx. It is measured during rest, squeeze, and straining. Normal values differ according to the method used. Perineal descent is present when the summit of the anorectal angle is below the level of the inferior ischial plane at rest or < 50mm on straining. In normal individuals, the resting level of the perineum descends with age, such that the extent of observed descent decreases with age. The level of the perineum is lower in women than in men and shows an association with the number of vaginal deliveries. The size of any rectocele is calculated during straining as the distance from the apex of the anterior rectal wall to a line drawn in the axis of the anal canal. As small rectoceles are frequently encountered in asymptomatic individuals, the finding of a rectocele is only considered to be of significance when it measures > 3cm in depth [32]. Circumferential intussusception is graded into four categories (1) fold thickness < 3mm (mucosal intussusception), (2) fold thickness > 3mm but not reaching the anal canal (rectorectal internal prolapse), (3) intra-anal (rectoanal internal prolapse), and (4) external prolapse. Absence of anorectal angle widening, and/or a prominent impression of the puborectalis sling during straining are signs of pelvic floor dyssynergia (puborectalis paradoxus). Rectal evacuation is recorded either subjectively on plain X-rays or extrapolated from plain views with specific programs. The orientation and movement of the other pelvic organs during defecation is also recorded. Caution must be taken to obtain radiographs before rectal filling, during straining, and after maximal rectal evacuation as rectal volume may impair the evaluation of other prolapses, such as an enterocele [33]. Peritoneography is used in some institutions to clarify any widening of the rectovaginal space. This widening may be due to an enterocele, or peritoneocele without enterocele. However, peritoneography improves diagnosis in only a very few patients with pelvic floor disorders and normal conventional defecography. Its routine use is limited by the necessary invasive puncture of abdominal wall.

In patients with ODS, the perineal position at rest is usually lower than in controls (Fig. 4.1). In patients with normal perineal position at rest, a greater degree of descent is frequently observed during straining compared to controls. Some patients with ODS may have an immobile perineum (< 1cm descent during straining). In these patients balloon expulsion is impaired, the anorectal angle does not widen, and distal colonic transit is abnormal.

Two types of rectocele are described: a distention (pulsion) type where anterior rectal distention is present in the absence of utero-vaginal prolapse

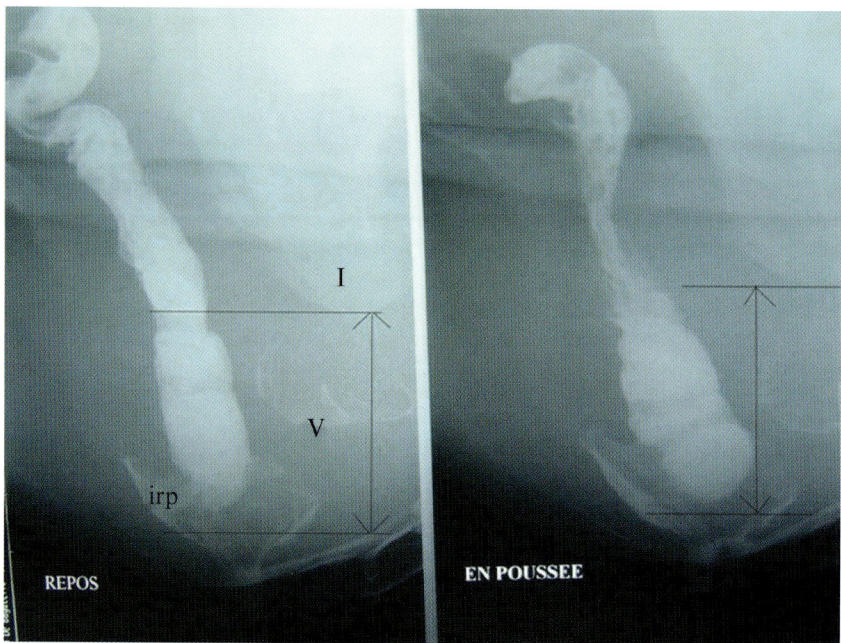

FIG. 4.1. X-ray defecography showing perineal descent with high-grade internal rectal prolapse (irp). Vagina (V). The perineal position is measured from the inferior edge of the ischial tuberosity (I) to the edge of the upper anal canal. The figure shows a normal perineal position (−60 mm) at rest (*left*) with little change (−65 mm) on straining (*right*)

(Fig. 4.2), and displacement type where rectocele formation follows the descent of a vaginal prolapse. Symptoms of constipation and colonic transit times, however, are similar in both types of rectocele. Puborectalis paradoxus is more frequently associated with the distension rectocele. In the displacement rectocele, anal resting and maximal contraction pressures are lower, the anorectal angle and perineal descent greater, and internal rectal prolapse more frequent [34]. Defecographic evidence of a rectocele correlated with a greater need to perform endovaginal digitation to initiate defecation, more frequent urogynecology symptoms, and a surgical history of hysterectomy [25, 35].

As a low-grade internal rectal prolapse is frequently found in asymptomatic individuals, significant internal rectal prolapse is defined as a fold thickness > 3mm with the apex of the prolapse reaching or penetrating the anal canal but not emerging through the anal verge, i.e., rectoanal internal prolapse (Fig. 4.3). Other classifications of rectal fold thickness and prolapse diameter have been proposed in an attempt to better distinguish symptomatic patients from controls [36]. Internal rectal prolapse may be found in patients with

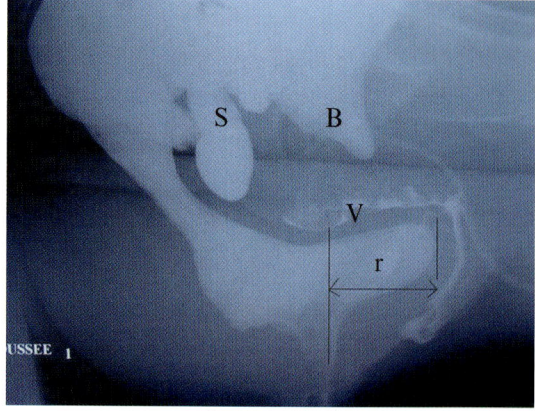

FIG. 4.2. X-ray defecography showing an isolated pulsion rectocele (r) during straining; small bowel (S), bladder (B), vagina (V)

ODS, independent of clinical symptoms. When rectal evacuation is incomplete on defecography, stasis is more frequently found in upper rectum compared to lower rectum stasis in patients with rectocele.

A peritoneocele is diagnosed when the peritoneum of the Pouch of Douglas extends below the

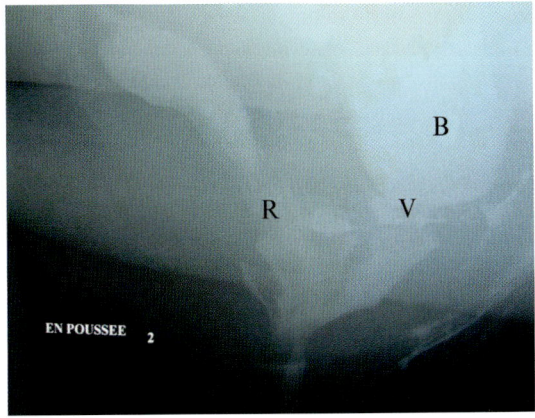

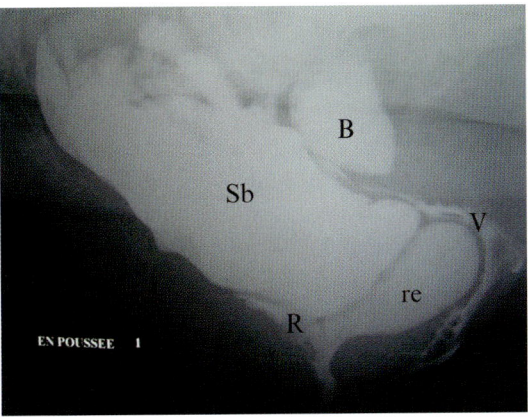

FIG. 4.3. X-ray defecography showing high-grade internal rectal prolapse (rectoanal) during straining; rectum (R), vagina (V), bladder (B)

FIG. 4.4. X-ray defecography showing an enterocele filled with small bowel loops (Sb) filling the rectovaginal space during straining; rectum (R) and rectocele (re), vagina (V), bladder (B)

level of the upper third of the vagina. Three types of peritoneocele are described according to their anteroposterior location: vaginal peritoneocele, septal peritoneocele, and rectal peritoneocele. An enterocele is diagnosed when small bowel is present within the peritoneal pouch, between the vagina and the rectum (Fig. 4.4). Enteroceles are more frequent in women with a past history of hysterectomy or cystopexy. They are rarely an isolated finding, being frequently associated with other pelvic organ prolapse. Sigmoidocele is a rare condition, sometimes found in patients with ODS.

The quantification of barium paste expelled during dynamic defecography may be subjectively evaluated from plain X-ray films, but has a poor reproducibility. Some authors recommend software extrapolation of rectal volumes taken from plain X-rays films. Rectal emptying is normal in 25% of patients with ODS [24]. In some reports, the presence of a rectocele has been associated with incomplete and prolonged rectal emptying on defecography and manometric evidence of anismus [24, 35]. Other reports have found no association between the presence of a rectocele and other defecographic measurements, the results of balloon expulsion tests, intrarectal pressure measurements, and the need for digitation [37, 38]. The need for vaginal digitation would appear to be more frequent in patients with a rectocele or anismus, as compared to intra-anal digitation which is more frequently encountered with internal rectal prolapse [39].

Dynamic Magnetic Resonance Imaging

The use of dynamic magnetic resonance imaging for the evaluation of pelvic floor dysfunction is growing in popularity. Prior to the MR imaging session, the patient's rectum is filled with contrast, for example 300ml of a synthetic stool consisting of potato starch mixed with 1.5ml of gadopentate dimeglumine (377mg/ml) (Magnevist®; Schering AG, Berlin, Germany), producing a gadolinium concentration of 2.5mmol/l. On the basis of localizing images in the axial, coronal, and sagittal planes, a multiphase fast T1-weighted spoiled gradient-recalled echo (SPGR) sequence is taken in the midsagittal plane of the anal canal with an image update every 2s.

Dynamic MRI has the advantage over contrast defecography in being a nonionizing radiological intervention and offering a more complete assessment of entire pelvic floor function. However, it is an expensive investigation, and critics point to the fact that defecation is simulated in a supine position on the MR table, which is unphysiological and makes it prone to the reporting of artifactual abnormalities. Despite these concerns, it is likely that the use of DMRI as a "one-stop" pelvic floor diagnostic tool will continue to expand.

Abnormalities of the pelvic floor are described in MR defecography in relation to the pubococcygeal line (PCL), a line joining the inferior border of the symphysis pubis to the last coccygeal joint in the midsagittal plane [40]. Descent of pelvic organs below the PCL is considered abnormal. Measurements are taken at the point of maximal displacement, which is usually at the end of defecation. The extent of any cystocele, enterocoele, anterior rectocele, or vaginal vault or rectal prolapse is measured at a 90° angle to the PCL and graded on a three-point scoring system as small, moderate, or large (Table 1) [41]. An anterior rectocele is defined as a protrusion of the rectal wall anterior to a line extending upward through the anal canal. The

size (depth) of an anterior rectocele is described as the depth of wall protrusion beyond the expected margin of the normal rectal wall and classified as small, moderate, or large (Table 1, Figs. 4.5 and 4.6) [40]. In addition, anterior rectoceles can be classified as those that empty completely with defecation and those which do not. Intussusception is classified into three grades: intrarectal (grade I), intra-anal (grade II), and external rectal prolapse (grade III).

TABLE 4.1. MR defecography grading system for pelvic floor pathology [26].

Abnormality	Small (cm)	Moderate (cm)	Large (cm)
Cystocele	< 3	3–6	> 6
Vaginal vault descent	< 3	3–6	> 6
Enterocele	< 3	3–6	> 6
Rectal descent	< 3	3–6	> 6
Anterior rectocele	< 2	2–4	> 4

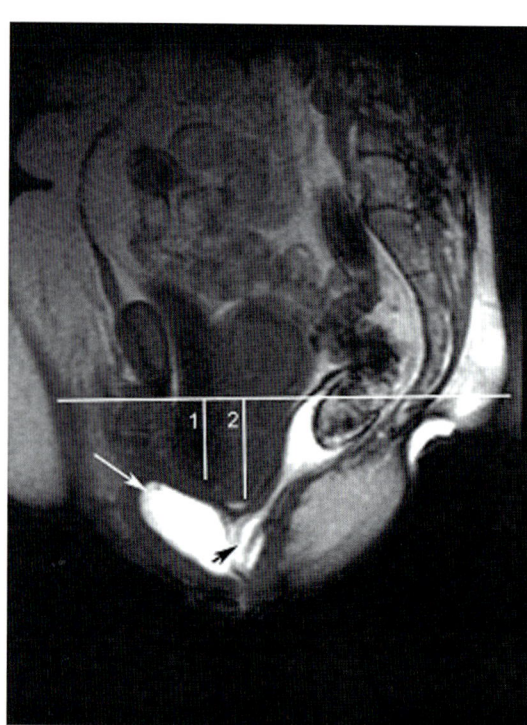

FIG. 4.5. Midsagittal MR images at rest, a moderate anterior rectocele (2.6 cm in sagittal diameter; *large white arrow*) as well as large rectal descent is noted (1, measurement for the posterior compartment).

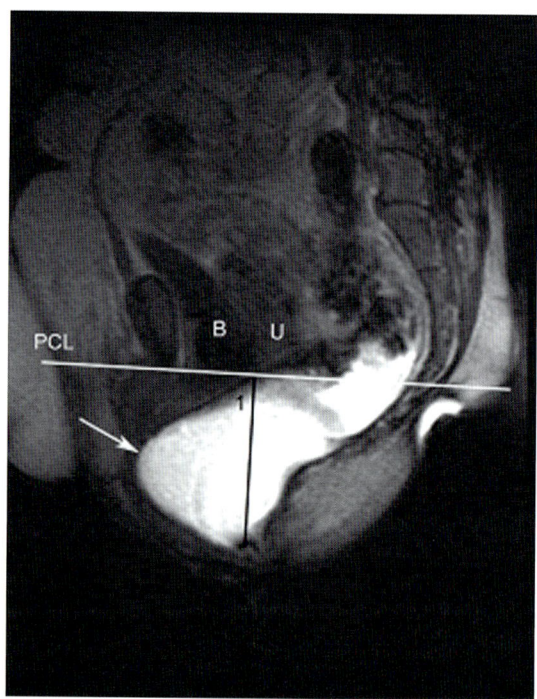

FIG. 4.6. At end of defecation, a large anterior rectocele (*large white arrow*) is present (4.8 cm in sagittal diameter) with incomplete evacuation of the contrast material (trapping). In addition, an internal prolapse is noted (*black small arrow*). The bladder base is located 3 cm (1) and the vaginal vault 3.6 cm (2) below the pubococcygeal line (PCL) consistent with a moderate cystocele and moderate vaginal vault descent. *B* Bladder, *U* Uterus

MRD appears to be at least equivalent to conventional defecography in terms of diagnostic yield. There is a suggestion that it might be less sensitive in detecting some abnormalities, such as minor degrees of intrarectal intussusception, while in other cases new findings of questionable significance have been described, including a widening of the puborectalis hiatus and an increased surface area of the levator muscles [42].

Measurement of Perineal Position with an External Plastic Cylinder

Attempts to quantify the extent of perineal descent have included the use of a graduated cylinder which is held against the anal verge and contained within a moving frame which in turn is pressed against the ischial tuberosities. Measurements are taken of the perineal position relative to the ischial tuberosities, both at rest and during a maximal straining effort [43]. It has limited value in routine clinical practice, producing results similar to those obtained from contrast defecography.

Electromechanical Rectal Barostat

Evaluation of rectal function with a barostat provides data on rectal compliance and visceral sensory perception. It is not a commonly used investigation, presently confined to the realms of surgical research.

Rectal compliance is known to decrease with age in normal individuals controls. It is abnormal in 20% of females with obstructed defecation and shows a strong association with the presence of a rectocele [44]. Abnormal rectal compliance may be secondary to an alteration in sympathetic and parasympathetic innervation, either primarily or secondary to chronic straining. The pressure thresholds for first sensation, earliest urge to defecate, and maximal tolerated volume are significantly higher in patients with obstructed defecation compared to controls [45, 46].

Endosonography

Most patients with ODS have similar sphincter anatomy to comparative controls on endoanal ultrasound (EAUS) examination. In a small subset of patients internal sphincter hypertrophy may be present and associated with anal hypertonia.

The main indication for EAUS is in the evaluation of coexistent sphincter dysfunction presenting as symptoms of fecal incontinence. Its routine use in patients with ODS and good sphincter function, as judged by a lack of incontinence symptoms and an intact sphincter and squeeze response on digital rectal examination, is debatable. Sphincter defects are found no more frequently than in controls, and may exist independent of symptoms of incontinence, or physiological evidence of sphincter dysfunction [47].

Advocates of EAUS have proposed its use as a nonionizing diagnostic modality for the detection of rectoceles, internal rectal prolapse, and enterocele [48]. It has also been suggested as a method for diagnosing anismus, with a distance of less than 5mm between the inner edge of the puborectalis muscle and the probe posteriorly, when measured at rest and on straining, being considered as pathological. In women with ODS, endosonography (either anal or vaginal) and perineal dynamic sonography were found to diagnose morphological and functional anomalies with a good concordance to conventional evaluation [49, 50].

Rectal Expulsion Tests

Introduced by Preston and Lennard-Jones in 1985 [51], rectal expulsion tests have been proposed to objectively quantify impaired rectal emptying in patients with symptoms of obstructed defecation.

Balloon expulsion is the simplest to perform. Different modifications of the test have been described which has hindered its standardization. It is most often performed with the patient in the left lateral position with a lubricated balloon inserted into the rectum. 50–60ml of water is injected into the balloon, and the patient is encouraged to make a maximum effort to expel it. If the balloon cannot be expelled in the left lateral position, the patient may sit on a modified commode, and the test repeated. Balloon volume may vary, with progressive filling until urge sensation is experienced. Expulsion may be facilitated with adding weights to the balloon. Normal controls are able to expel a 50-ml balloon in the left lateral position. A positive evacuation test is not specific of ODS; although it is abnormal in 50–80% of patients with ODS, evacuation tests may also be abnormal in 50% of patients with simple constipation [52, 53].

It has been suggested that expulsion of a balloon filled with 60ml air/liquid in patients without any rectal anatomical defect (such as rectocele or internal rectal prolapse) might be useful in selecting patients with pelvic floor dyssynergia [54].

Some authors have proposed viscous fluid expulsion as being representative of normal physiological conditions. Instant weighting of evacuated paste or isotopic defecometry may then be used to evaluate evacuation flow rate [55].The viscous fluid expulsion test has a reported sensitivity of 100% and a specificity of 82% in patients with ODS, when compared with retention of contrast on dynamic defecography, suggesting that mechanisms other than anatomical defects may be responsible for symptoms of ODS [53].

Fecoflowmetry gives an indication of the rate of paste evacuation and can be combined with simultaneous registration of anal and rectal pressures. It distinguishes normal transit constipation and obstructed defecation [55]. Although promising, this test has not been validated in other institutions.

Electromyographic Studies

Electromyographic studies give information on the quality of motor innervation and synchronization during straining or voiding efforts. Different recording techniques (surface, concentric needle, and single-fiber electrodes) have been validated. At rest the pelvic floor musculature normally remains in a state of continuous activity. The fiber density within the external anal sphincter muscle is determined using single-fiber EMG. The normal fiber density is 1.5 ± 0.16 and increases slightly after 65 years of age. Recordings of motor unit potentials are made with the patient at rest, during voluntary contraction of the external sphincter, and during simulated defecation. During straining a coordinated inhibition of the puborectalis muscle and external anal sphincter muscle should occur.

Pudendal nerve terminal motor latency (PNTML) measurements are made via a rubber finger stall having two stimulating electrodes at its tip and two surface electrodes for recording at its base. With the device placed on the index finger and inserted into the rectum the pudendal nerve is stimulated transrectally at the level of the ischial spine and the latency of the response in the external anal sphincter muscle recorded by the surface electrode

is measured on the EMG graph. The mean terminal motor latency is 2.0 ± 03ms.

Needle perineal electromyography (fasiculations and fibrillation) and pudendal nerve terminal motor latency (prolonged neuronal conduction) give information about motor nerve fiber denervation. It must be stressed that the frequency of neuropathy increases with age, both in the normal population and in patients with defecatory disorders.

Pudendal neuropathy is found in one-fourth patients with constipation, independent of sex or pelvic floor dyssynergia [56]. Repeated straining efforts are thought to give rise to perineal trauma and neuropathy resulting in perineal descent [57]. The degree of neuropathy positively correlates with the age of the patient and the extent of perineal descent [58].

Other neurogenic alterations, in addition to motor neuropathies, may be found in patients with ODS. Sensory pudendal neuropathy may be demonstrated by an increased electric and thermal sensitivity threshold in anal canal and rectum in patients with dyschezia compared to controls [59]. Anal mucosal hyposensitivity to electrical stimulation is found in 20% of female patients with constipation, uncorrelated with rectal hyposensity to volumetric balloon distension [60]. Mechanisms involved in these neurological anomalies may be due to diffuse alterations in the enteric nervous system, rather than a sole pudendal neuropathy.

A lack of decrease of electrical activity during maximal straining effort has long been considered a function of pelvic floor dyssynergia. However, EMG findings do not always correlate with the ability to evacuate the rectum, with symptoms of obstructed defecation, or with other tests for pelvic floor dyssynergia.

Pelvic Floor Dyssynergia (Anismus, Nonrelaxing Puborectalis Syndrome, Pelvic Floor Dysfunction)

Pelvic floor dyssynergia (PFD) is defined as paradoxical contraction or failure to relax the pelvic floor striated muscles (external anal sphincter and puborectalis) during attempts to defecate. According to the Rome criteria [61], the following must be present:

1. Clinical evidence of functional constipation
2. Paradoxical perineal contraction or absence of relaxation demonstrated by at least two of the following tests: manometry, electromyography, or defecography
3. Evidence of adequate intrarectal propulsive forces
4. Incomplete rectal emptying.
5. PFD may be one of many causes for ODS, which includes inadequate stool propulsion through the colon into the rectum, impaired perception of stool in the rectum, uncoordinated rectal contraction, poor straining ability, and failure of reflex relaxation of the internal sphincter, and external sphincter/puborectalis muscle [23].

Many tests may be used to demonstrate inadequate coordination of the perineal muscles during straining: defecography shows an insufficient increase ($< 5\%$) in the anorectal angle on straining, and/or persistence of the puborectalis indentation on posterior rectal wall; manometry reveals an absence of anal pressure reduction; and EMG shows an increased or insufficient inhibition ($< 20\%$) of electrical activity of the external sphincter/puborectalis (exploration with concentric or fine-wire needles may be done in either the external sphincter or puborectalis as they act in the same manner) [63].

However, none of these tests is specific for pelvic floor dyssynergia as they are frequently positive in asymptomatic controls (20–60%) and in patients with other anorectal symptoms such as incontinence (10–70%) and perineal pain (40–50%) [63, 64]. One explanation could be the nonphysiological conditions in which the tests are performed, giving rise to heightened levels of patient stress. In patients with constipation, with or without ODS, pelvic floor dyssynergia is reported anywhere between 20 and 80%.

Agreement between the various tests for pelvic dyssynergia is poor, with correlation being found in less than one-third of patients. Furthermore, the results depend on the methods of testing. For example, EMG diagnosis of anismus is influenced by patient position and rectal filling volume, and might diminish when the patient is seated and the rectum is filled with contents [65, 66]. Furthermore, agreement with intrarectal balloon expulsion testing is also poor. It is possible that these different tests evaluate a different aspect of rectal function, such that expulsion tests reflect more the ability to increase rectal pressure rather than the synchronization of pelvic musculature during the straining effort [51, 55].

The significance of pelvic floor dyssynergia is important when found in patients without an obvious rectal anatomical defect. The first-line treatment for these patients is biofeedback rehabilitation in an attempt to correct the uncoordinated pelvic floor contraction. The significance of dyssynergia in patients with anomalies such as rectocele, or high-grade internal rectal prolapse is controversial. Some regard the dyssynergia as the primary etiology underlying the ODS, with the anatomical abnormalities being a secondary phenomenon. As such, the presence of dyssynergia is regarded as a poor prognostic indicator for rectocele repair. Others regard dyssynergia as merely part of the disease process and not necessarily a contraindication to surgical intervention.

As no clinical symptom is specific for PFD, and as diagnosis relies on a combination of more than one abnormal test, the laboratory evaluation may be extensive and expensive. Selection of patients on simple clinical criteria may be of value. In two series, the negative predictive value of normal digital examination, or balloon expulsion test was 82% and 97%, respectively [54, 66].

Predictive Factors for Therapeutic Intervention

In women with ODS, significant perineal descent at rest associated with a low voluntary anal canal squeeze pressure were predictive factors for anal incontinence [21].

The traditional treatment for patients with PFD is biofeedback rehabilitation, with reported success rates ranging widely between 20–80%. As outcome is independent of the presence of rectocele or internal prolapse [69], it is suggested that patients with rectal static disorders and PFD should undergo biofeedback trial before surgery. The results after biofeedback therapy appear to be influenced by the type of PFD encountered. Two types of defecographic anismus are described:

1. *Type A*. flattened anorectal angle, without puborectalis indentation, but a closed canal anal
2. *Type B*. A clear puborectalis indentation, narrow anorectal angle and closed canal anal
3. Type A PFD has poorer results after biofeedback [70]. Some authors have suggested that biofeedback rehabilitation should also be the preferred

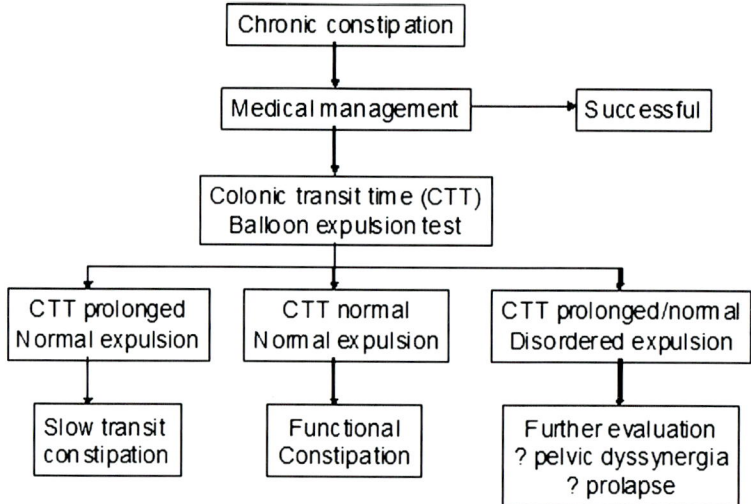

FIG. 4.7. proposed diagnostic algorithm for constipated patients

first-line treatment in patients with ODS in the absence of PFD [71, 72].

In a series of patients operated on for an internal rectal prolapse by Delorme's procedure, preoperative criteria for poor outcome included proximal internal rectal prolapse with rectosacral separation and descending perineum of more than 9 cm on defecography, chronic diarrhea, and incontinence [73]. Among 76 patients operated transanally for ODS and rectocele and/or anterior rectal wall prolapse, a larger preoperative volume at which urge to defecate was elicited was a good predictor of continence improvement and resolution of obstructive defecation. Neither the defecography size of the rectocele nor anal pressures were predictive of functional results after surgery [74]. Pelvic floor dyssynergia has been described as a negative predictive factor for outcome following rectocele surgery [75], but indifferent in others [76].

Conclusion

Clinical history and examination remains the mainstay for diagnosing and clinical decision making in patients with symptomatic hemorrhoids. It is clearly important to exclude other colorectal pathology, and at the very least a rigid sigmoidoscopy or

endoscopic examination of the left colon should be undertaken with the exception of perhaps the young patient without other worrying symptoms. Further radiological and physiological investigation should be reserved for those patients in whom hemorrhoidal symptoms coexist with symptoms of other pelvic floor dysfunction or in whom there is concern regarding the functional integrity of the anal sphincter.

In contrast, all patients presenting with constipation and obstructed defecation require extensive investigation to classify the nature of the disease process and to assess coexistent pelvic floor pathology. Only when this has been determined can the patient be appropriately advised regarding the most appropriate form of treatment. A proposed diagnostic algorithm for patients presenting with constipation is presented in Fig. 4.7

References

1. Mehanna D, Platell C. Investigating chronic, bright red, rectal bleeding. ANZ J Surg 2001;71:720–722
2. Cheung PSY, Wong SKC, Boey J, Lai CK. Frank rectal bleeding: a prospective study of causes in patients over the age of 40. Postgraduate Med J 1988;64:364–368
3. Gibbons CP, Bannister JJ, Read NW. Role of constipation and anal hypertonia in the pathogenesis of haemorrhoids. Br J Surg 1988;75:656–660

4. Sun WM, Read NW, Shorthouse AJ. Hypertensive anal cushions as a cause of the high anal canal pressures in patients with haemorrhoids. Br J Surg 1990;77:458–462

5. Bruck CED, Lubowski DZ, King DW. Do patients with haemorrhoids have pelvic floor denervation? Int J Colorect Dis 1988;3:210–214

6. Read NW, Bartolo DCC, Read MG, Hall J, Haynes WG, Johnson AG. Differences in ano-rectal manometry between patients with haemorrhoids and patients with descending perineum syndrome: implications for management. Br J Surg 1983;70:656–659

7. Champigneulle B, Dieterling P, Bigard MA, Gaucher P. Etude prospective de la fonction sphinctérienne anale avant et après hémorroïdectomie. Gastroenterol Clin Biol 1989;13:452–456

8. Ho YH, Tan M. Ambulatory anorectal manometric findings in patients before and after haemorrhoidectomy. Int J Colorect Dis 1997;12:296–297

9. Patti R, Almasio PL, Arcara M, Sparacello M, Termine S, Bonventre S, Di Vita G. Long-term manometric study of anal sphincter function after hemorrhoidectomy. Int J Colorectal Dis 2007;22:253–257

10. Read MG, Read NW, Haynes WG, Donnelly TC, Johnson AG. A prospective study of the effect of haemorrhoidectomy on sphincter function and faecal continence. Br J Surg 1982;69:396–398

11. Bursics A, Weltner J, Flautner LE, Morvay K. Anorectal physiological changes after rubber band ligation and closed haemorrhoidectomy. Colorectal Dis 2004;6:58–61

12. Chauhan A, Thomas S, Bishnoi PK, Hadke NS. Randomized controlled trial to assess the role of raised anal pressures in the pathogenesis of symptomatic early hemorrhoids. Dig Surg. 2007;24:28–32

13. Abbasakoor F, Nelson M, Beynon J, Patel B, Carr ND Anal endosonography in patients with anorectal symptoms after haemorrhoidectomy. Br J Surg 1998;85:1522–1524

14. Felt-Bersma RJ, van Baren R, Koorevaar M, Strijers RL, Cuesta MA. Unsuspected sphincter defects shown by anal endosonography after anorectal surgery. A prospective study. Dis Colon Rectum 1995;38:249–253

15. Boccasanta P, Venturi M, Roviaro G. Stapled transanal rectal resection versus stapled anopexy in the cure of hemorrhoids associated with rectal prolapse. A randomized controlled trial. Int J Colorectal Dis 2007;22:245–251

16. Ho YH, Seow-Choen F, Goh HS. Haemorrhoidectomy and disordered rectal and anal physiology in patients with prolapsed haemorrhoids. Br J Surg 1995;82:596–598

17. Halverson AL, Orkin BA. Which physiologic tests are useful in patients with constipation? Dis Colon Rectum 1998;41:735–739

18. Knowles CH, Eccersley AJ, Scott SM, Walker SM, Reeves B, Lunniss PJ. Linear discriminant analysis of symptoms in patients with chronic constipation: validation of a new scoring system (KESS). Dis Colon Rectum 2000;43:1419–1426

19. Koch A, Voderholzer WA, Klauser AG, Müller-Lissner S. Symptoms in chronic constipation. Dis Colon Rectum 1997;40:902–906

20. Rasmussen OO, Sorensen M, Tetzschner T, Christiansen J. Dynamic anal manometry in the assessment of patients with obstructed defecation. Dis Colon Rectum 1993;36:901–907

21. Berkelmans I, Heresbach D, Leroi AM, Touchais JY, Martin PA, Weber J, Denis P. Perineal descent at defecography in women with straining at stool: a lack of specificity or predictive value for future anal incontinence? Eur J Gastroenterol Hepatol 1995;7:75–79

22. Ducrotte P, Rodomanska B, Weber J, Guillard JF, Lerebours E, Hecketsweiler P, Galmiche JP, Colin R, Denis P. Colonic transit time of radiopaque markers and rectoanal manometry in patients complaining of constipation. Dis Colon Rectum 1986;29:630–634

23. Rao SS, Welcher KD, Leistikow JS. Obstructive defecation: a failure of rectoanal coordination. Am J Gastroenterol 1998;93:1042–1050

24. Siproudhis L, Le Gall R, Ropert A, Reignier A, Heresbach D, Raoul JL, Renet C, Bretagne JF, Gosselin M.Does manometric megarectum have a symptomatic role in patients complaining of dyschezia? Gastroenterol Clin Biol 1993;17:162–167

25. Siproudhis L, Ropert A, Lucas J, Raoul JL, Heresbach D, Bretagne JF, Gosselin M. Defecatory disorders, anorectal and pelvic floor dysfunction: a polygamy? Radiologic and manometric studies in 41 patients. Int J Colorectal Dis 1992;7:102–107

26. Dinning PG, Bampton PA, Andre J, Kennedy ML, Lubowski DZ, King DW, Cook IJ. Abnormal predefecatory colonic motor patterns define constipation in obstructed defecation. Gastroenterology 2004;127:49–56

27. Preston DM, Lennard-Jones JE, Thomas BM. Towards a radiologic definition of idiopathic megacolon. Gastrointest Radiol 1985;10:167–169

28. Chaussade S, Khyari A, Roche H, Garret M, Gaudric M, Couturier D, Guerre J. Determination of total and segmental colonic transit time in constipated patients. Dis Colon Rectum 1989;34:1168–1172

29. Ahran P, Devroede G, Jehannin B, Lanza M, Faverdin C, Dornic C, Persoz B, Tetrault L, Peret B, Pellerin D. Segmental colonic transit time. Dis Colon Rectum 1981;24:625–629

30. Grotz RL, Pemberton JH, Talley NJ, Rath DM, Zinsmeister AR. Discriminant value of psychological distress, symptom profiles, and segmental

colonic dysfunction in outpatients with severe idiopathic constipation. Gut 1994;35:798–802

31. Mahieu P, Pringot J, Bodart P. Defecography: II. Contribution to the diagnosis of defecation disorders. Gastrointets Radiol 1984;9:253–261

32. Shorvon PJ, Mc Hugh S, Diamant NE, Somers S, Stevenson GW. Defecography in normal volunteers: results and implications. Gut 1989;30:1737–1749

33. Bremmer S, Mellgren A, Holmstrom B, Uden R. Pelvic anatomy and pathology is influenced by distention of the rectum: defecoperitoneography before and after rectal filling with contrast medium. Dis Colon Rectum 1997;40:1477–1483

34. Pucciani F, Rottoli ML, Bologna A, Buri M, Cianchi F, Pagliai P, Cortesini C. Anterior rectocele and anorectal dysfunction. Int J Colorectal Dis 1996;11:1–9

35. Siproudhis L, Ropert A, Vilotte J, et al. How accurate is clinical examination in diagnosing and quantifying pelvirectal disorders ? A prospective study in a group of 50 patients complaining of defecatory difficulties. Dis Colon rectum 1993;36:430–438

36. Pomerri F, Zuliani M, Mazza C, Villarejo F, Scopece A. Defecographic measurements of rectal intussusception and prolapse in patients and in asymptomatic subjects. Am J Roentgol 2001;176:641–645

37. Wald A, Caruana BJ, Freimanis MG, Bauman DH, Hinds JP. Contributions of evacuation proctography and anorectal manometry to evaluation of adults with constipation and defecatory difficulty. Dig Dis Sci 1990;35:481–487

38. Halligan S, Bartram CI. Is barium trapping in rectoceles significant? Dis Colon Rectum 1995;38:764–768

39. Halligan S, Bartram CI. Is digitation associated with proctographic abnormality? Int J Colorectal Dis 1996;11:167–171

40. Roos JE, Weishaupt D, Wildermuth S, Willmann JK, Marincek B, Hilfiker PR. Experience of 4 years with the open MR defecography: pictorial review of anorectal anatomy and disease. Radiographics 2002;22:817–832

41. Kelvin FM, Maglinte DD, Hale DS, Benson JT. Female pelvic organ prolapse: a comparison of triphasic dynamic MR imaging and triphasic fluoroscopic cystocoloproctography. AJR 2000;174:81–88

42. Healy JC, Halligan S, Reznek RH, Watson S, Bartram CI, Kamm MA, Phillips RK, Armstrong P. Magnetic resonance imaging of the pelvic floor in patients with obstructed defaecation. Br J Surg 1997;84:1555–1558

43. Henry MM, Parks AG, Swash M. The pelvic floor musculature in the descending perineum syndrome. Br J Surg 1982;69:470–472

44. Gosselink MJ, Hop WC, Schouten WR. Rectal compliance in females with obstructed defecation. Dis Colon Rectum 2001;44:971–977

45. Schouten WR, Gosselink MJ, Boerma MO, Ginai AZ. Rectal wall contractility in response to an evoked urge to defecate in patients with obstructed defecation. Dis Colon Rectum 1998;41:473–479

46. Gosselink MJ, Schouten WR. Rectal sensory perception in females with obstructed defecation. Dis Colon Rectum 2001;44:1337–1344

47. Nielsen MB, Rasmussen OO, Pedersen JF, Christiansen J. Anal endosonographic findings in patients with obstructed defecation. Acta Radiol 1993;34:35–38

48. Karaus M, Neuhaus P, Wiedenmann TB. Diagnosis of enteroceles by dynamic anorectal endosonography. Dis Colon Rectum 2000;43:1683–1688

49. Murad-Regadas SM, Regadas FS, Rodrigues LV, Silva FR, Soares FA, Escalante RD. A novel three-dimensional dynamic anorectal ultrasonography technique (echodefecography) to assess obstructed defecation, a comparison with defecography. Surg Endosc 2007;20 (in press)

50. Brusciano L, Limongelli P, Pescatori M, Napolitano V, Gagliardi G, Maffettone V, Rossetti G, Del Genio G, Russo G, Pizza F, Del Genio A. Ultrasonographic patterns in patients with obstructed defaecation. Int J Colorectal Dis 2007;22:969–77

51. Preston DM, Lennard-Jones JE. Anismus in chronic constipation. Dig Dis Sci 1985;30:413–418

52. Alstrup N, Ronholt C, Fu C, Rasmussen O, Sorensen M, Christiansen J. Viscous fluid expulsion in the evaluation of the constipated patient. Dis Colon Rectum 1997;40:580–584

53. Papachrysostomou M, Smith AN, Merrick MV. Obstructive defaecation and slow transit constipation: the proctographic parameters. Int J Colorectal Dis 1994;9:115–120

54. Minguez M, Herreros B, Sanchiz V, Hernandez V, Almela P, Añon R, Mora F, Benages A. Predictive value of the balloon expulsion test for excluding the diagnosis of pelvic floor dyssynergia in constipation. Gastroenterology 2004;126:57–62

55. Shafik A, Abdel-Moneim K. Fecoflowmetry: a new parameter assessing rectal function in normal and constipated patients. Dis Colon Rectum 1993;36:35–42

56. Vaccaro CA, Wexner SD, Teoh TA, Choi SK, Cheong DM, Salanga VD. Pudendal neuropathy is not related to physiologic pelvic outlet obstruction. Dis Colon Rectum 1995;38:630–634

57. Kiff ES, Barnes PR, Swash M. Evidence of pudendal neuropathy in patients with perineal descent and chronic straining at stool. Gut 1984;25:1279–1282

58. Engel AF, Kamm MA. The acute effect of straining on pelvic floor neurological function. Int J Colorectal Dis 1994;9:8–12

59. Solana A, Roig JV, Villoslada C, Hinojosa J, Lledo S. Anorectal sensitivity in patients with obstructed defaecation. Int J Colorectal Dis 1996;11:65–70

60. Vasudevan SP, Scott SM, Gladman MA, Lunniss PJ. Rectal hyposensitivity: evaluation of anal sensation in female patients with refractory constipation with and without faecal incontinence. Neurogastroenterol Motil 2007;19:660–667

61. Whitehead WE, Wald A, Diamant NE, Enck P, Pemberton JH, Rao SSC. Functional disorders of the anus and rectum. Gut 1999;45:1155–1159

62. Fucini C, Ronchi O, Elbetti C. Electromyography of the pelvic floor musculature in the assessment of obstructed defecation symptoms. Dis Colon Rectum 2001;44:1168–1175

63. Schouten WR, Briel JW, Auwerda JJ, van Dam JH, Gosselink MJ, Ginai AZ, Hop WC. Anismus: fact or fiction? Dis Colon Rectum 1997;40:1033–1041

64. Jones PN, Lubowski DZ, Swash M, Henry MM. Is paradoxical contraction of puborectalis muscle of functional importance? Dis Colon Rectum 1987;30:667–670

65. Lopez A, Holmstrom B, Nilsson BY, Dolk A, Johansson C, Schultz I, Zetterstrom J, Mellgren A. Paradoxical sphincter reaction is influenced by rectal filling volume. Dis Colon Rectum 1998;41:1017–1022

66. Karlbom U, Edebol Eeg-Olofsson K, Graf W, Nilsson S, Pahlman L. Paradoxical puborectalis contraction is associated with impaired rectal evacuation. Int J Colorectal Dis 1998;13:141–147

67. Halligan S, Thomas J, Bartram C. Intrarectal pressures and balloon expulsion related to evacuation proctography. Gut. 1995;37:100–104

68. Schouten WR, Briel JW, Auwerda JJ, van Dam JH, Gosselink MJ, Ginai AZ, Hop WC. Anismus: fact or fiction? Dis Colon Rectum 1997;40:1033–1041

69. Lau C-W, Heymens S, Alabaz O, Iroatulam AJN, Wexner SD. Prognsotic significance of rectal intussusception, and abnormal perineal descent in biofeedback treatment for constipated patients with paradoxical puborectalis contraction. Dis Colon Rectum 2000;43:478–482

70. Park UC, Choi SK, Piccirillo MF, Verzaro R, Wexner SD. Patterns of anismus and the relation to biofeedback therapy. Dis Colon Rectum 1996;39:768–773

71. Karlbom U, Hallden M, Eeg-Olofsson KE, Pahlman L, Graf W. Results of biofeedback in constipated patients: a prospective study. Dis Colon Rectum 1997;40:1149–1155

72. Ho YH, Tan M, Goh HS. Clinical and physiologic effects of biofeedback in outlet obstruction constipation. Dis Colon Rectum 1996;39:520–524

73. Sielezneff I, Malouf A, Cesari J, Brunet C, Sarles JC, Sastre B. Selection criteria for internal rectal prolapse repair by Delorme' transrectal excision. Dis Colon Rectum 1999;42:367–373

74. Janssen LW, van Dijke CF. Selection criteria for anterior rectal wall repair in symptomatic rectocele and anterior rectal wall prolapse. Dis Colon Rectum 1994;37:1100–1107

75. Tjandra JJ, Ooi BS, Tang CL, Dwyer P, Carey M. Transanal repair of rectocele corrects obstructed defecation if it is not associated with anismus. Dis Colon Rectum 1999;42:1544–1550

76. van Dam JH, Hop WC, Schouten WR. Analysis of patients with poor outcome of rectocele repair. Dis Colon Rectum 2000;43:1556–1560

Chapter 5
Patient Selection for Stapled Hemorrhoidopexy and STARR

Oliver Schwandner and Roland Scherer

Abstract Stapled hemorrhoidopexy using the PPH-stapling device aims to resect and reduce the volume of prolapsing hemorrhoidal tissue and to restore it to its normal anatomical position within the anal canal. In contrast, the STARR procedure aims to produce a full-thickness resection of the lower rectum, removing the distal rectal redundancy which may manifest as a rectocele and/or internal rectal prolapse, alleviating symptoms of obstructed defecation. Currently, two staplers and two techniques exist for the performance of STARR. Like any surgical intervention, the success of stapled hemorrhoidopexy and STARR is related to careful patient selection. This chapter sets out the principles involved in patient selection for stapled hemorrhoidopexy and STARR and defines the appropriate indications and contraindications for each procedure.

Patient Selection for Stapled Hemorrhoidopexy

Indications for Stapled Hemorrhoidopexy

The treatment of hemorrhoids is based on the degree of prolapse in conjunction with associated symptoms. The Goligher classification of hemorrhoids remains the most widely used [1]: first-degree hemorrhoids bleed but do not prolapse; second-degree hemorrhoids prolapse on straining to defecate and reduce spontaneously; third-degree hemorrhoids prolapse on straining but can be reduced manually; and fourth-degree hemorrhoids are permanently prolapsed and cannot be manually reduced. Internal hemorrhoids may cause pruritis (anal itching and irritation), bleeding, and soiling. They may prolapse outside the anus causing a palpable or visible swelling. Although anal discomfort is frequently a presenting complaint, acute pain is not a typical symptom. If pain is a predominant symptom then consideration should be given to the existence of other pathologies such as anal fissure, intersphincteric abscess, or proctitis, which are usually readily diagnosed on clinical examination. Stapled hemorrhoidopexy is indicated for patients suffering with symptomatic hemorrhoidal prolapse, i.e., symptoms due to Goligher grade II–IV hemorrhoids.

In 2007 the National Institute for Health and Clinical Excellence published its updated guidance on stapled hemorrhoidopexy [2]. This stated "Stapled haemorrhoidopexy, using a circular stapler specifically developed for haemorrhoidopexy, is recommended as an option for people in whom surgical intervention is considered appropriate for the treatment of prolapsed internal haemorrhoids." The guidance did not give any specific recommendations as to the indications or contraindications for stapled hemorrhoidopexy. It considered 27 randomized controlled trials comparing stapled hemorrhoidopexy with either Milligan–Morgan or Ferguson hemorrhoidectomy. This cohort included a mixed cohort of patients suffering with grade II to IV hemorrhoidal prolapse.

Assessment of the literature regarding stapled hemorrhoidopexy and grade of prolapse is not the

D. Jayne and A. Stuto (eds.), *Transanal Stapling Techniques for Anorectal Prolapse*, DOI: 10.1007/978-1-84800-905-9_5, © Springer-Verlag London Limited 2009

remit of this chapter and is discussed in greater detail in Chaps. 8 and 9. It is sufficient to note that interpretation of the literature is made difficult by heterogeneity of the data. Many studies have compared stapled hemorrhoidopexy with Milligan–Morgan hemorrhoidectomy or Ferguson's closed hemorrhoidectomy. Most of these studies have included patients with third- and fourth-degree hemorrhoids [3–18]. Other studies have included patients with second-degree hemorrhoids [11, 19–25], and two studies have restricted investigation to patients with fourth-degree hemorrhoids [26, 27]. In some studies there has been no clear definition regarding patient selection and degree of prolapse [4, 21, 22, 28–30]. From this mix of data, the following are regarded as generally accepted principles among surgeons practicing hemorrhoidopexy.

First-degree piles, which do not prolapse, can be readily treated by dietary modification, or if necessary by nonexcisional methods, and should not be considered for stapled hemorrhoidopexy.

Most second-degree hemorrhoids are amenable to either dietary modification or nonexcisional methods, such as injection sclerotherapy, rubberband ligation, or infrared coagulation. Only when nonexcisional methods have failed should hemorrhoidectomy be considered. However, stapled hemorrhoidopexy may considered as first-line therapy in patients with circumferential grade II hemorrhoids, where the number of rubber bands needed to be applied for adequate reduction of the prolapse is likely to be prohibitive. However, it should be noted that the evidence supporting the use of stapled hemorrhoidopexy in grade II prolapse is limited.

It is in the treatment of grade III hemorrhoids that stapled hemorrhoidopexy appears to be particularly advantageous. Most trials of stapled hemorrhoidopexy for grade III prolapse have shown long-term outcomes at least as good as conventional hemorrhoidectomy with the added benefits of reduced postoperative pain, shorter hospital stay, and earlier return to normal function. The limited cost-effectiveness data that are available also suggests that the cost of the stapler is likely to be offset by the shorter hospital stay and quicker recovery [2].

The use of stapled hemorrhoidopexy in grade IV prolapse is more controversial. A prerequisite to its use is that the hemorrhoidal prolapse should be reducible under anesthesia. Although it is safe

and probably as effect as conventional hemorrhoidectomy in the short term, there is a recognized increased incidence of recurrent prolapse on long-term follow-up [2, 27, 31]. The possible reasons for this are discussed in greater detail in Chap. 9. It would appear that the higher incidence of recurrent prolapse is related to insufficient prolapse resection produced by the stapler in large volume hemorrhoidal disease. It is important to appreciate that some 16% of patients presenting with hemorrhoidal prolapse will have symptoms of obstructed defecation [32] and may have associated internal rectal prolapse or rectocele. In these patients, a stapled hemorrhoidopexy, although dealing with the hemorrhoidal prolapse, will do nothing for the internal rectal prolapse, which will be the cause of recurrent symptoms. Thus, all patients presenting with hemorrhoidal prolapse should be specifically questioned regarding associated symptoms of obstructed defecation. If these exist, then further investigation by means of defecating proctography is indicated. If internal rectal prolapse is identified it may be that the patient is best suited to either a double-stapled PPH technique [33] or a modified STARR procedure [34].

The routine use of stapled hemorrhoidopexy in acute hemorrhoidal prolapse and thrombosis cannot be recommended, although Brown et al. have demonstrated its feasibility with reasonable results, albeit with very limited follow-up [26].

In practical terms the categorization of hemorrhoidal prolapse into four distinct categories is somewhat artificial. Often patients present with a mixture of third- and fourth-degree prolapse or third-degree with skin tags giving the appearance of fourth-degree prolapse. The issue of associated skin tags should not really alter the proposed management. Rarely are skin tags so large that conventional hemorrhoidopexy would be preferred over stapled hemorrhoidopexy. Any associated skin tags can either be left in situ if they are not troublesome, or can be safely dealt with by simple excision on completion of the stapling procedure without added morbidity. There will inevitably be some increased postoperative discomfort following excision of skin tags, but it is still likely to be less painful than a three-pedicle hemorrhoidectomy. The authors' preference is to excise any large skin tags at the same time as stapled hemorrhoidopexy, accepting a degree of increased postoperative discomfort but avoiding the need for reintervention. Despite anecdotal reports of skin tags naturally reducing in size following stapled hemorrhoidopexy, they rarely resolve completely and can remain a source of anal irritation. Residual skin tags may also be misinterpreted by patients for recurrent prolapse [9], and for this reason they are usually best removed at the time of stapled hemorrhoidopexy.

Contraindications for Stapled Hemorrhoidopexy

There are few contraindications to performing stapled hemorrhoidopexy. Those that exist have been previously documented in a 2003 consensus paper produced by an international working party [35]. For practical purposes they are considered below as absolute and relative contraindications.

Absolute Contraindications

- Situations where stapled hemorrhoidopexy is technically not feasible:
  - Patients with anal stenosis

- Situations where stapled hemorrhoidopexy is technically feasible, but potentially dangerous for the patient. These include the presence of coexistent anorectal disease:

  - Anal sepsis, abscess, or fistula
  - Anal or rectal cancer or other tumors
  - Intra-anal condylomata
  - Acute proctitis due to inflammatory bowel disease, radiotherapy, etc.
  - Anorectal sexually transmitted diseases

Relative Contraindications

- Situations where stapled hemorrhoidopexy is technically feasible, but may be unnecessary or result in a suboptimal outcome:

  - First-degree hemorrhoids
  - Fixed, not reducible fourth-degree hemorrhoids

- Situations where stapled hemorrhoidopexy is technically feasible, but maybe difficult with a high risk of complications:

  - Previous low rectal or coloanal anastomosis
  - Previous proctological surgery resulting in rigidity of the anorectum

  - Previous sphincter reconstruction
  - Patients with known or potential bleeding disorders, e.g., anticoagulant medication, liver cirrhosis, renal failure
  - Patients at risk of septic complications as a result of transient bacteremia, e.g., immunosuppressed patients, patients undergoing chemotherapy, HIV patients

- Situations where stapled hemorrhoidopexy is technically possible, but may be dangerous for the partner:

  - Patients (male or female) practicing receptive anal intercourse

Special Considerations

A group of patients where stapled hemorrhoidopexy may be of particular benefit is those suffering with liver cirrhosis and portal hypertension [36–38]. Although the risks of bleeding will be higher than in noncirrhotic patients, this may be reduced with stapled hemorrhoidopexy as compared to conventional hemorrhoidectomy. In addition, the avoidance of open anal wounds has the theoretical advantage of reduced local sepsis and associated portal pyemia.

Any patients practicing receptive anal intercourse should be warned of the dangers of the staple line causing penile injury or condom rupture in the early postoperative period [39, 40]. Such patients should be advised to refrain from anal penetration until such time as all the staples have fallen out. This usually takes between 3 and 6 weeks, although isolated staples may remain embedded indefinitely.

Patient Selection for STARR

Internal rectal prolapse (rectal intussusception) and rectocele are frequent findings in patients suffering from Obstructive Defecation Syndrome (ODS). They are considered to be manifestations of an underlying redundancy of the distal rectum, which on straining to defecate acts as an obstruction to rectal evacuation. The STARR procedure aims to resect the distal rectal redundancy resulting in a neorectum which is straightened and resuspended, allowing normalization of defecation (Fig. 5.1).

The short-term safety and efficacy of STARR for obstructed defecation has been documented

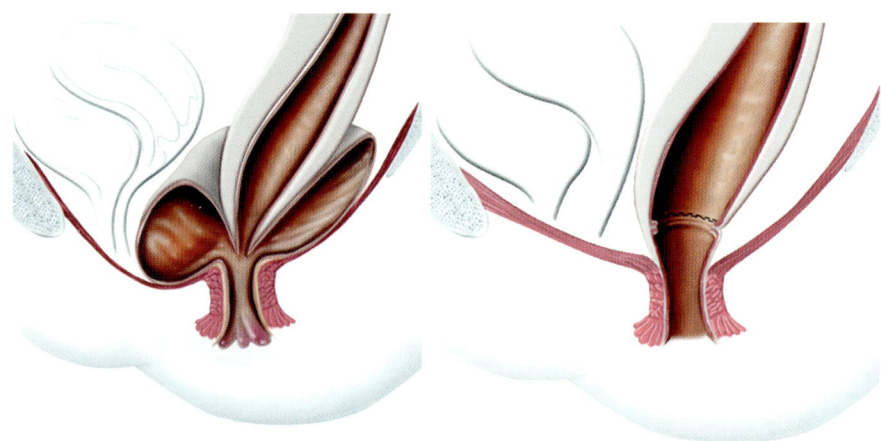

Fig. 5.1. Stapled transanal rectal resection (STARR): the distal rectal redundancy with rectocele and internal prolapse is resected with simultaneous anastomosis to produce a straightened neo-rectum

in various studies [41–44] (See Chap. 8 for literature review). However, some case reports have highlighted the potential for serious complications which have been the focus for concern [45, 46]. To date, there is still no clear evidence regarding the long-term efficacy of STARR [47, 48].

The reporting of adverse outcomes related to STARR probably relates to poor patient selection as much as poor surgical technique. Although the indications for STARR in terms of ODS and internal rectal prolapse have been defined, ODS is in fact a symptom complex which may be associated with one or more underlying pathologies. It may result from either a functional pelvic floor problem (dyssynergia), a definable anatomical abnormality (internal prolapse with or without rectocele) or a combination of the two. In addition, in some 30–40% of cases, ODS and internal rectal prolapse may coexist with anatomical abnormalities and prolapse of the middle and anterior pelvic compartments. Thus to consider posterior (rectal) compartment prolapse in isolation as an indication for STARR is likely to result in unpredictable outcomes.

From a technical point of view, the STARR may be considered as an extension of the PPH procedure for hemorrhoids. Certainly, the surgeon should be competent with stapled hemorrhoidopexy before considering progressing to STARR. However, STARR involves a circumferential

full-thickness resection of the lower rectum and as such is technically much more challenging. Although the double-stapled PPH STARR can be mastered with relative ease, the Contour30 (Transtar) involves a stapling technique distinct from any other colorectal procedure. The learning curve with the Contour30 (Transtar) has not been defined, and it is recommended that it should not be undertaken prior to adequate training and preceptorship.

Of paramount importance when assessing patients for STARR is the need to take a thorough clinical history. This should focus on symptoms of ODS, but include a full obstetric and urogynecological history. Only those patients with symptoms suggestive of ODS (listed later) should be subjected to further investigation. It is helpful to quantify ODS symptoms by means of a scoring system, either that proposed by Longo or one of its modifications [49]. Although the ODS score will give an indication of the severity of the symptoms, it should not be used as an indicator for surgical intervention. In the past, predefined ODS scores of > 9 or >12 have been used in clinical trials as a cut-off for STARR [50]. However, the ODS score is not a predictor of outcome and should not be used for this purpose. Its value is as a comparator to assess efficacy before and after treatment and to compare patient cohorts in terms of disease severity between different clinical studies.

Definition of ODS

ODS may be defined as the normal desire to defecate, but an impaired ability to satisfactorily evacuate the rectum. Typical symptoms include:

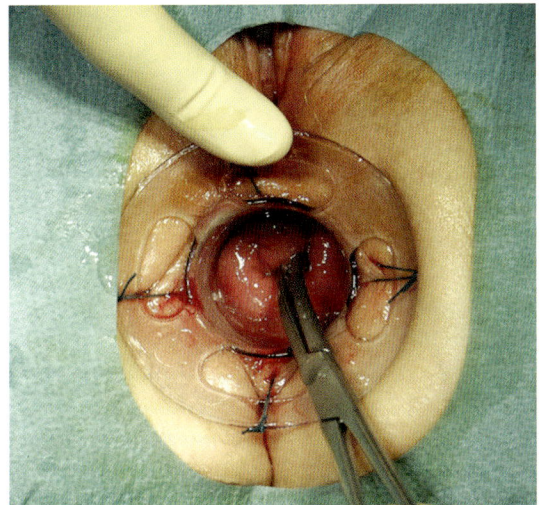

FIG. 5.2. Internal rectal prolapse as demonstrated at operation

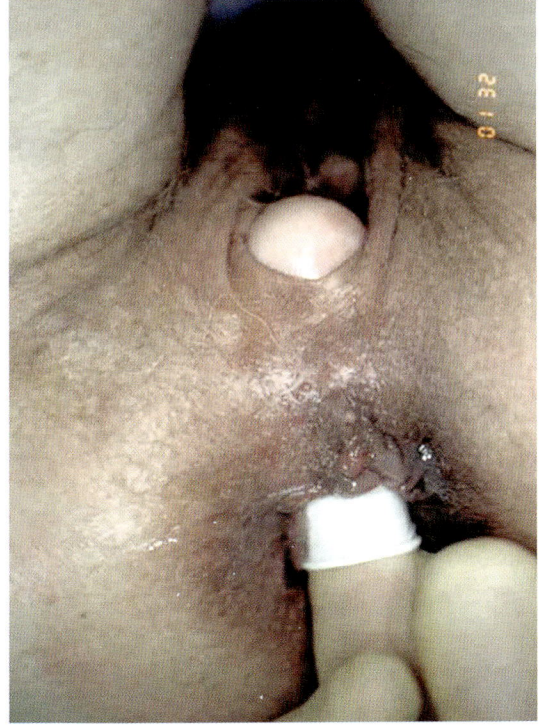

FIG. 5.3. Anterior rectocele as demonstrated at operation

- Prolonged or repeated straining to achieve defecation
- An excessive time spent on the toilet to achieve defecation
- A sense of incomplete rectal evacuation
- Frequent calls to defecate
- Use of digital manipulation or perineal support to initiate evacuation
- A dependency on regular laxatives or enemas
- Pelvic pressure, rectal discomfort, and perineal pain

Clinical examination frequently reveals the presence of an internal rectal prolapse and/or an anterior rectocele (Figs. 5.2 and 5.3). Patients with a good history of ODS and detectable redundancy of the distal rectum on clinical examination should be offered further investigation to determine their suitability for STARR or other treatment modality.

Diagnostic Assessment and Patient Selection for STARR

Careful and thorough diagnostic assessment is essential in all patients being considered for STARR. It is mandatory to exclude colorectal malignancy and inflammatory bowel disease, preferably by colonoscopy. Dynamic radiological imaging either by contrast defecography or dynamic MRI is recommended in all patients to establish and categorize any structural abnormalities of the rectum and pelvic floor. The use of routine anal manometry and endoanal ultrasound is more contentious if digital rectal examination has shown a normal anal sphincter. However, it is essential in patients with a history of fecal incontinence, urgency, or suspected anal sphincter injury. It is also useful in clarifying the diagnosis in patients with suspected pelvic dyssynergia (anismus, paradoxical puborectalis syndrome).

Many clinicians would recommend a course of conservative treatment for all patients with ODS prior to undertaking surgical intervention [51]. This might include a combination of dietary manipulation, defecatory regulation with enemas and laxatives, pelvic floor retraining, biofeedback, or colonic irrigation. The chorology to this view is that most patients, by the time they are seen by a coloproctologist, have already tried a variety of medical treatments and they are seeking a surgical solution to their problem. In addition, the results of best medical management, including biofeedback therapy, are unimpressive with symptomatic response in only ~50% of patients ODS and rectocele [52] and ~30% of patients with ODS and intussusception [51]. As a consequence, many proctologists are now taking the view that if the patient has good symptoms of ODS and a demonstrable redundancy of the distal rectum then the STARR procedure should be considered as first-line treatment.

Treatment Options After Dynamic Imaging with Special Reference to the STARR Procedure

Like any other surgical intervention, patient selection for STARR is crucial to a satisfactory outcome. It cannot be overemphasized that the presence of a rectocele or internal rectal prolapse in the absence of ODS symptoms is not an indication for STARR. Or, put another way, STARR is not advocated as a surgical correction for rectocele and internal rectal prolapse in the absence of ODS symptoms.

The following treatment algorithm is suggested as a guide to therapeutic intervention based on the results of diagnostic assessment:

(a) *ODS with isolated internal rectal prolapse.* In patients with a good history of ODS and evidence of distal rectal redundancy, either in the form of rectocele and/or internal prolapse, the STARR procedure can be recommended as the initial treatment option. This assumes that other pelvic floor pathologies have been excluded and that the patient has normal anal sphincter function (Fig. 5.4).

(b) *ODS and internal rectal prolapse in the presence of other anatomical pelvic floor abnormalities.* In patients with ODS and internal rectal prolapse who have other anatomical pelvic floor abnormalities, such as enterocele, sigmoidocoele, or urogenital prolapse, treatment of these associated disorders is recommended in the first instance (Fig. 5.5). This is likely to involve a multidisciplinary approach with a gynecologist who has an interest in pelvic floor dysfunction. Once associated pelvic floor problems have

been corrected, if symptoms of ODS persist then recourse to a STARR as a secondary intervention might be considered to deal with the any residual internal rectal prolapse. If an enterocele is encountered in the presence of internal rectal prolapse, it is reasonable to approach the problem with a combination of laparoscopy and STARR: the enterocoele is reduced laparoscopically and the laparoscope kept in place to provide views of the pelvis while the STARR is performed [53]. This protects the small bowel from inadvertent injury. Provided STARR achieves an adequate full-thickness resection, the low-lying pouch of Douglas will be closed, obliterating the peritoneal sac and dealing with the enterocele. Similarly, in the presence of a significant sigmoidocele, consideration may be given to performing a laparoscopic sigmoid resection in combination with a STARR. If this is to be undertaken, it is preferable to preserve the superior rectal vessels for fear of leaving an ischemic rectal segment between the sigmoid resection above and the STARR resection below.

(c) *ODS and internal rectal prolapse in the presence of pelvic floor dyssynergia.* Patients with ODS and internal rectal prolapse who are found to have coexistent pelvic dyssynergia (anismus, spastic pelvic floor, puborectalis paradoxus) are unlikely to achieve a successful outcome if treated by STARR in the first instance. These patients should be offered pelvic floor retraining with biofeedback therapy (Fig. 5.6). With further experience it is possible that a subset of these patients may be shown to derive some benefit from STARR, but currently in these conditions STARR cannot be recommended.

(d) *ODS and internal rectal prolapse in the presence of poor anal sphincter function.* In patients with ODS and internal rectal prolapse who have a history of incontinence or documented poor sphincter function on anorectal physiology testing then one should proceed with caution (Fig. 5.7). In such cases the defecatory urgency, which affects 15–20% of patients following STARR, is likely to exacerbate pre-existing incontinent symptoms. The same is true in patients with a hypersensitive rectum, as demonstrated by low threshold and maximal tolerated volumes on balloon distension, and those patients with a tendency to diarrhea (diarrhea predominant irritable bowel syndrome). If STARR is to be performed in the presence of poor anal sphincter function, then the patient should be appropriately warned of the increased risk of defecatory urgency and possible incontinence. Some reassurance may be given that any urgency associated with STARR is likely to be transient, resolving by 3–6 months postoperatively and may be responsive to the use of antidiarrheal medications.

In patients with coexistent anal sphincter dysfunction a tailored approach taking into consideration the predominant symptom, either constipation or incontinence, is often the best way forward. In a proportion of patients, symptoms of incontinence will be attributable to the internal rectal prolapse particularly if intra-anal intussusception is demonstrated on defecating proctography. In these patients, resection of the internal rectal prolapse will lead to

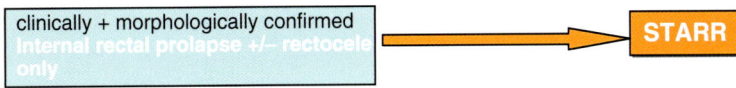

FIG. 5.4. Treatment options in "classical" ODS due to internal prolapse alone

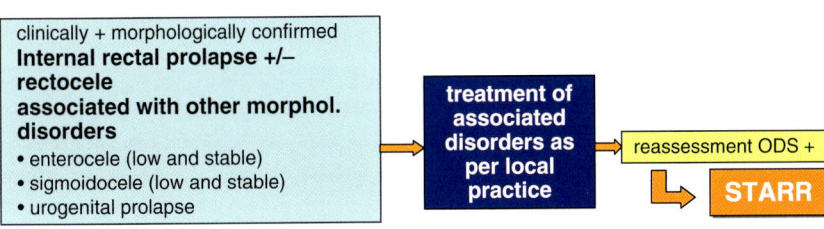

FIG. 5.5. Treatment options if internal prolapse is associated with additional morphological disorders

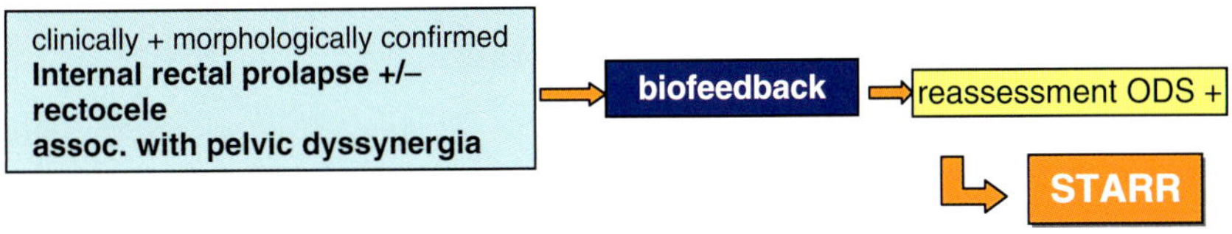

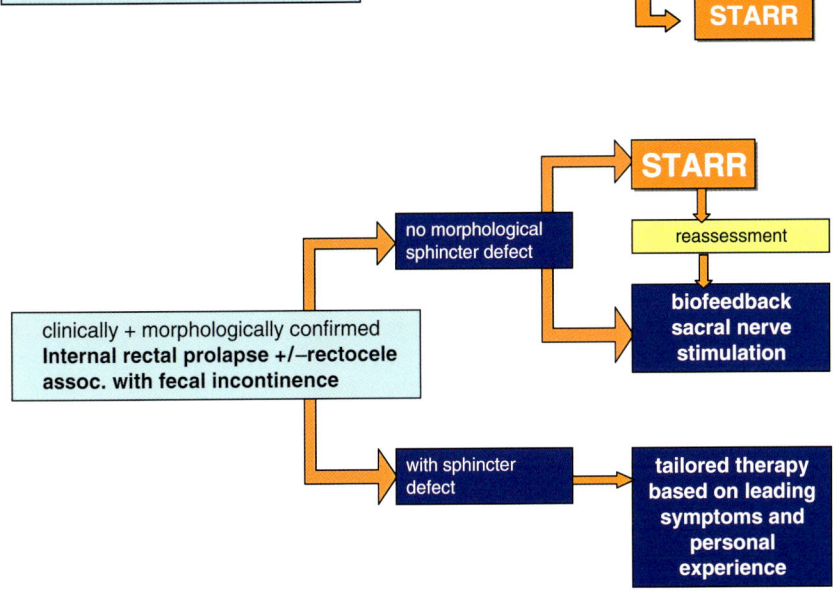

FIG. 5.6. Treatment options in ODS with pelvic dyssynergy

FIG. 5.7. Treatment options if internal prolapse is associated with fecal incontinence

both correction of the ODS and an improvement in continence. Unfortunately, there is as yet no discriminative test to enable the clinician to judge the likely outcome at the preoperative stage. Should STARR result in intractable defecatory urgency or incontinence uncontrollable with antidiarrheal agents, then consideration should be given to performing a sphincteroplasty if a discrete anatomical sphincter defect exists or to sacral nerve modulation. In patients with a documented sphincter defect, it is not advised to attempt a sphincteroplasty as the first procedure. This is likely to exacerbate ODS symptoms, which will no longer be amenable to STARR for fear of disruption of the repaired sphincter.

Contraindications for STARR

The following absolute and relative contraindications for STARR have been suggested, based on the collective experience and recommendations from the 2006 STARR consensus meeting [47] and the 2008 position statement created by the STARR Pioneer group [54].

Absolute contraindications to STARR:

- Active anorectal sepsis (abscess, fistula, etc.)
- Concurrent anorectal pathology, including anal stenosis
- Proctitis (inflammatory bowel disease, radiation proctitis)
- Enterocele at rest (low and stable)
- Chronic diarrhea

Relative exclusion criteria include:

- Presence of foreign material adjacent to the rectum (e.g., prosthetic mesh from a previous rectocele repair or pelvic floor resuspension)
- Previous anterior resection or transanal surgery with rectal anastomosis
- Concurrent psychiatric disorder

In general, the contraindications for STARR include any condition which might predispose to postoperative sepsis (abscess, fistula) or make the resection technically difficult due to the presence of an inflamed and thickened rectal wall which will not readily prolapse into the stapler (proctitis for any cause, previous implanted prosthetic mesh, previous transanal surgery).

For the purposes of patient selection for STARR, enteroceles can be classified into those which are low lying and stable (present at rest on defecography) and those that are dynamic and only appear on straining to defecate. Generally, STARR can be performed safely in patients with a dynamic enterocele provided that bimanual examination of the rectum and vagina at the time of surgery excludes the presence of an enterocele, and sufficient head-down tilt of the operating table is used to exclude the small bowel from the pelvis. If there is any doubt, it is recommended that a laparoscope be inserted and the small bowel retracted out of the pouch of Douglas prior to performing STARR. This strategy may also be successful in cases with a low-lying, stable enterocele.

Patients with suspected irritable bowel syndrome should be fully evaluated using the standardized Rome II or III criteria [55]. As yet, the results of STARR in patients with irritable bowel syndrome are unknown, and prudence is recommended particularly if diarrheal symptoms predominate. Patients with constipation-predominant irritable bowel may benefit from STARR provided they fulfill the other criteria for intervention.

A prior history of anterior resection was previously considered to be an absolute contraindication for STARR for fear of producing an ischemic segment of rectum. Experience, although limited, suggests that this is more of a relative contraindication. Provided there is no associated peripheral vascular disease and a sufficient length of time has passed following anterior resection, then it is probably safe to undertake STARR. Similarly, it appears to be safe to perform STARR as a redo procedure following a previously inadequate outcome, or to treat recurrence after other transanal techniques (internal Delorme's, sutured rectopexy, etc.). When undertaking STARR for recurrent disease it should be anticipated that it will be technically more demanding as a result of residual mesorectal fibrosis.

Patients with coexistent psychological or psychiatric disorders should be carefully assessed prior to advising STARR [56]. A formal assessment by a psychologist or a psychiatrist is valuable to determine the extent of any nonorganic cause for their defecatory problems and to review any psychiatric medications which might be exacerbating their symptoms. However, patients should not automatically be refused STARR based on a psychiatric history alone. Many patients with ODS have a history of chronic, severe defecatory dysfunction going back over many years, which may well have contributed to an obsessional preoccupation with their bowels. In addition, there has been a tendency in the past for members of the medical profession to label patients with chronic defecatory problems as being "mad." This probably results from their own poor understanding of the etiology underlying ODS and the lack of a good surgical solution.

In patients with multicompartment pelvic floor dysfunction, including urogential prolapse and external rectal prolapse, it is unlikely that the STARR procedure will provide symptom resolution when performed in isolation (Fig. 5.8). These patients require assessment in a combined pelvic floor clinic with input from a urogynecologist, coloproctologist, pelvic floor physiotherapist, etc. to determine the best treatment strategy. If external rectal prolapse exists in isolation, modifications of the STARR procedure have been proposed, but experience is limited and as yet this approach cannot be recommended as evidence-based.

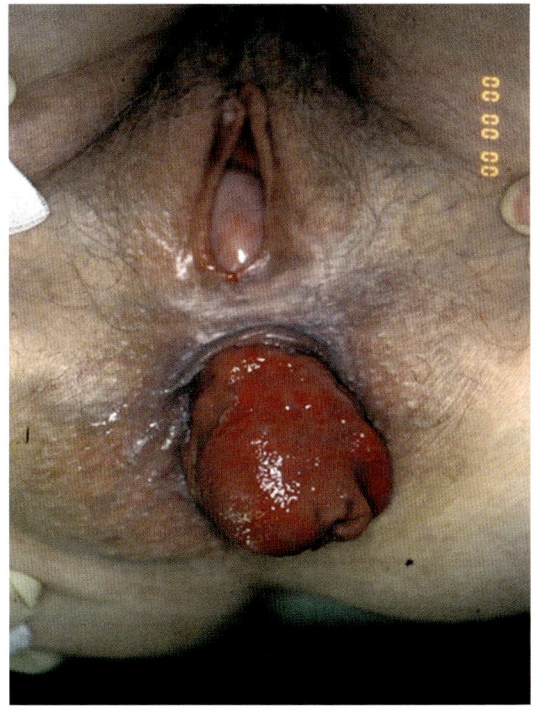

FIG. 5.8. Multicompartment pelvic floor failure with genital prolapse and external rectal prolapse

Summary

Stapled hemorrhoidopexy is recommended as a treatment option for symptomatic prolapsing piles. It may be useful in grade II prolapse which have failed to respond to nonexcisional therapies. The evidence would suggest it is of maximal benefit in grade III and IV hemorrhoidal prolapse, although the recurrent prolapse rate appears to be higher if the volume of hemorrhoidal disease is large. The absolute and relative contraindications to stapled hemorrhoidopexy are outlined.

The STARR procedure is indicated in patients with ODS associated with redundancy of the distal rectum as manifest by rectocele and/or internal rectal prolapse. When considering patients for STARR it is important to consider ODS as a complex, multifactorial condition which is commonly associated with other pelvic floor pathologies. A combined multidisciplinary approach is often necessary. A treatment algorithm for STARR is provided.

References

1. Goligher JC. Surgery of the anus, rectum and colon. 5th ed. London: Bailliere Tindall; 1984
2. National Institute for Health and Clinical Excellence. Stapled haemorrhoidopexy for the treatment of haemorrhoids: NICE technology appraisal guidance 128, 2007
3. Palimento D, Picchio M, Attanasio U, Lombardi A, Bambini C, Renda A. Stapled and open hemorrhoidectomy: randomized controlled trial of early results. World J Surg 2003; 27: 203–207
4. Smyth EF, Baker RP, Wilken BJ, Hartley JE, White TJ, Monson JR. Stapled versus excision haemorrhoidectomy: long-term follow up of a randomised controlled trial. Lancet 2003; 361: 1437–1438
5. Wilson MS, Pope V, Doran HE, Fearn SJ, Brough WA. Objective comparison of stapled anopexy and open hemorrhoidectomy: a randomized, controlled trial. Dis Colon Rect 2002; 45: 1437–1444
6. Kanellos I, Angelopoulos S, Zacharakis E, Kanellos D, Pramateftakis MG, Blouhos K, et al. Stapled haemorrhoidopexy for haemorrhoids in combination with lateral internal sphincterotomy for fissure-in-ano. Eur Surg Res 2005; 37: 317–320
7. Maw A, Concepcion R, Eu KW, Seow-Choen F, Heah SM, Tang CL, et al. Prospective randomized study of bacteraemia in diathermy and stapled haemorrhoidectomy. Br J Surg 2003; 90: 222–226

8. Ho YH, Seow-Choen F, Tsang C, Eu KW. Randomized trial assessing anal sphincter injuries after stapled haemorrhoidectomy. Br J Surg 2001; 88: 1449–1455

9. Ganio E, Altomare DF, Gabrielli F, Milito G, Canuti S. Prospective randomized multicentre trial comparing stapled with open haemorrhoidectomy. Br J Surg 2001; 88: 669–674

10. Senagore AJ, Singer M, Abcarian H, Fleshman J, Corman M, Wexner S, et al. A prospective, randomized, controlled multicenter trial comparing stapled hemorrhoidopexy and Ferguson hemorrhoidectomy: perioperative and one-year results. Dis Colon Rect 2004; 47: 1824–1836

11. Thaha MA, Irvine LA, Steele RJ, Campbell KL. Postdefaecation pain syndrome after circular stapled anopexy is abolished by oral nifedipine. Br J Surg 2005; 92: 208–210

12. Rowsell M, Bello M, Hemingway DM. Circumferential mucosectomy (stapled haemorrhoidectomy) versus conventional haemorrhoidectomy: randomised controlled trial. Lancet 2000; 355: 779–781

13. Basdanis G, Papadopoulos VN, Michalopoulos A, Apostolidis S, Harlaftis N. Randomized clinical trial of stapled hemorrhoidectomy vs open with Ligasure for prolapsed piles. Surg Endoscopy 2005; 2: 235–239

14. Kairaluoma M, Nuorva K, Kellokumpu I. Day-case stapled (circular) vs. diathermy hemorrhoidectomy: a randomized, controlled trial evaluating surgical and functional outcome. Dis Colon Rect 2003; 46: 93–99

15. Chung CC, Cheung HY, Chan ES, Kwok SY, Li MK. Stapled hemorrhoidopexy vs. Harmonic Scalpel hemorrhoidectomy: a randomized trial. Dis Colon Rect 2005; 48: 1213–1219

16. Longman RJ, Thomson WH. A prospective study of outcome from rubber band ligation of piles. Colorectal Dis 2006; 8: 145–148

17. Kirsch JJ, Staude G, Herold A. The Longo and Milligan–Morgan hemorrhoidectomy. A prospective comparative study of 300 patients. Chirurg 2001; 72: 180–185

18. Lan P, Wu X, Zhou X, Wang J, Zhang L. The safety and efficacy of stapled hemorrhoidectomy in the treatment of hemorrhoids: a systematic review and meta-analysis of ten randomized control trials. Int J Colorectal Dis 2006; 21: 172–178

19. Pavlidis T, Papaziogas B, Souparis A. Modern stapled Longo procedure vs. conventional Milligan–Morgan hemorrhoidectomy: a randomized controlled trial. Int J Colorectal Dis 2002; 17: 50–53

20. Hetzer FH, Demartines N, Handschin AE, Clavien PA. Stapled vs excision hemorrhoidectomy: long-term results of a prospective randomized trial. Arch Surg 2002; 137: 337–340

21. Cheetham MJ, Cohen CR, Kamm MA, Phillips RK. A randomized, controlled trial of diathermy hemorrhoidectomy vs. stapled hemorrhoidectomy in an intended day-care setting with longer-term follow-up. Dis Colon Rect 2003; 46: 491–497

22. Shalaby R, Desoky A. Randomized clinical trial of stapled versus Milligan–Morgan haemorrhoidectomy. Br J Surg 2001; 88: 1049–1053

23. Khalil KH, O'Bichere A, Sellu D. Randomized clinical trial of sutured versus stapled closed haemorrhoidectomy. Br J Surg 2000; 87: 1352–1355

24. Van de SJ, D'Hoore A, Duinslaeger M, Chasse E, Penninckx F. Belgian Section of Colorectal Surgery Royal Belgian Society for Surgery. Long-term results after excision haemorrhoidectomy versus stapled haemorrhoidopexy for prolapsing haemorrhoids; a Belgian prospective randomized trial. Acta Chirurgica Belgica 2005; 105: 44–52

25. Lau PY, Meng WC, Yip AW. Stapled haemorrhoidectomy in Chinese patients: a prospective randomised control study. Hong Kong Med J 2004; 10: 373–377

26. Brown SR, Seow-Choen F. Stapled mucosectomy for acute throbosed circumferentially prolapsed piles: a prospective randomized comparison with conventional haemorrhoidectomy. Colorectal Dis 2001; 3: 175–178

27. Ortiz H, Marzo J, Armendariz P, de MM. Stapled hemorrhoidopexy vs. diathermy excision for fourth-degree hemorrhoids: a randomized, clinical trial and review of the literature. Dis Colon Rect 2005; 48: 809–815

28. Au-Yong I, Rowsell M, Hemingway DM. Randomised controlled clinical trial of stapled haemorrhoidectomy vs conventional haemorrhoidectomy; a three and a half year follow up. Colorectal Dis 2004; 6: 37–38

29. Gravie JF, Lehur PA, Huten N, Papillon M, Fantoli M, Descottes B, et al. Stapled hemorrhoidopexy versus milligan-morgan hemorrhoidectomy: a prospective, randomized, multicenter trial with 2-year postoperative follow up. Ann Surg 2005; 242: 29–35

30. Picchio M, Palimento D, Attanasio U, Renda A. Stapled vs open hemorrhoidectomy: long-term outcome of a randomized controlled trial. Int J Colorectal Dis 2006; 21: 668–669

31. Ortiz H, Marzo J, Armendariz P. Randomized clinical trial of stapled haemorrhoidopexy versus conventional diathermy haemorrhoidectomy. Br J Surg 2002; 89: 1376–1381

32. Schwandner O, Bruch HP. Significance of obstructed defaecation in haemorrhoidal disease: results of a prospective study. Coloproctol 2006; 28: 13–20

33. Papagrigoriadis S, Vardonikolaki A. Stapled anopexy with double stapling: a safe and efficient treatment for fourth degree haemorrhoids. Acta Chirurgica Belgica 2006; 106: 717–718

34. Boccasanta P, Venturi M, Gaincario R. Stapled transanal rectal resection versus stapled anopexy in the cure of hemorrhoids associated with rectal prolapse. A randomised controlled trial. Int J Colorectal Dis 2007; 22: 245–251

35. Corman ML, Gravie JF, Hager T, Loudon MA, Mascagni D, Nystrom PO, et al. Stapled haemorrhoidopexy: a consensus position paper by an international working party – indications, contraindications and technique. Colorectal Dis 2003; 5: 304–310

36. Huang WS, Lin PY, Chiu CC, Yeh CH, Hsieh CC, Chuang TS, et al. Stapled hemorrhoidopexy for prolapsed hemorrhoids in patients with liver cirrhosis, a preliminary outcome of 8-case experience. Int J Colorectal Dis 2007; 22: 1083–1089

37. Hegedus L, Ladocsi B, Wellner I, Olah A. New surgical method in the treatment of severe hemorrhoidal bleeding caused by decompensated liver cirrhosis. Magyar Sebeszet 2001; 54: 52–53

38. Parvaiz A, Azeem S, Singh RK, Lamparelli M. Stapled hemorrhoidopexy: an alternative technique for the treatment of bleeding anorectal varices. Report of a case. Dis Colon Rect 2006; 49: 411–412

39. Mlakar B. Should we avoid stapled hemorrhoidopexy in males and females who practice receptive anal sex? Dis Colon Rect 2007; 50: 1727

40. Kekez T, Bulic K, Smudj D, Majerovic M. Is stapled hemorrhoidopexy safe for the male homosexual patient? Report of a case. Surg Today 2007; 37: 335–337

41. Boccasanta P, Venturi M, Stuto A, Bottini C, Caviglia A, Carriero A, et al. Stapled transanal rectal resection for outlet obstruction: a prospective, multicenter trial. Dis Colon Rectum 2004; 47: 1285–1297

42. Schwandner O, Farke S, Bruch HP. Stapled transanal rectal resection (STARR) for obstructed defecation caused by rectocele and rectoanal intussusception. Viszeralchirurgie 2005; 40: 331–341

43. Ommer A, Albrecht K, Wenger F, Walz MK. Stapled transanal rectal resection (STARR): a new option in the treatment of obstructive defecation syndrome. Langenbeck's Arch Surg 2006; 391: 32–37

44. Schwandner O, Fürst A. German STARR Registry (2007) Preliminary results of a prospective, multicenter observational study. Coloproctol 2007; 29: 13–21

45. Pescatori M, Dodi G, Salafia C, Zbar AP. Rectovaginal fistula after double-stapled transanal rectotomy (STARR) for obstructed defecation. Int J Colorectal Dis 2005; 20: 83–85

46. Dodi G, Pietroletti R, Milito G, Binda G, Pescatori M. Bleeding, incontinence, pain and constipation after STARR transanal double stapling rectotomy for obstructed defecation. Tech Coloproctol 2003; 7: 148–153

47. Corman ML, Carriero A, Hager T, Herold A, Jayne DG, Lehur PA, et al. Consensus conference on the stapled rectal resection resection (STARR) for disordered defaecation. Colorectal Dis 2006; 8: 98–101

48. Jayne DG, Finan PJ. Stapled transanal rectal resection for obstructed defaecation and evidence-based practice. Br J Surg 2005; 92: 793–794

49. Altomore DF, Spazzafuma L, Rinaldi M, Dodi G, Ghiselli R, Piloni V. Set-up and statistical validation of a new scoring system for obstructed defaecation syndrome. Colorectal Dis 2008; 10: 84–88

50. Renzi A, Izzo D, Di Sarno G, Izzo G, Di Martino N. Stapled transanal rectal resection to treat obstructed defecation caused by rectal intussusception and rectocele. Int J Colorectal Dis 2006; 21: 661–667

51. Choi JS, Hwang YH, Salum MR, Weiss EG, Pikarsky AJ, Nogueras JJ, et al. Outcome and management of patients with large rectoanal intussusception. Am J Gastroenterol 2001; 96: 740–744

52. Mimura T, Roy AJ, Storrie JB, Kamm MA. Treatment of impaired defecation associated with rectocele by behavioral retraining (biofeedback). Dis Colon Rect 2000; 43: 1267–1272

53. Petersen S, Hellmich G, Schuster A, Lehmann D, Albert W, Ludwig K. Stapled transanal rectal resection under laparoscopic surveillance for rectocele and concomitant enterocele. Dis Colon Rectum 2006; 49: 1–5

54. Schwandner O, Stuto A, Jayne D, Lenisa L, Pigot F, Tuech JJ, Scherer R, Nugent K, Corbisier F, Basany EE, Hetzer FH. Decision-making algorithm for the STARR procedure in obstructed defecation syndrome: position statement of the group of STARR pioneers. Surg Innov 2008; 15: 105–109 DOI 10.1177/1553350608316684

55. Sperber AD, Shvartzman P, Friger M, Fich A. A comparative reappraisal of the Rome II and Rome III diagnostic criteria: are we getting closer to the "true" prevalence of irritable bowel syndrome? 1. Eur J Gastroenterol Hepatol 2007; 19: 441–447

56. Renzi C, Pescatori M. Psychologic aspects in proctalgia. Dis Colon Rectum 2000; 43: 535–539

Chapter 6
Stapled Hemorrhoidopexy: The Technique

E. Espin and F. Corbisier

Abstract Stapled hemorrhoidopexy is indicated for the treatment of symptomatic prolapsing piles. Although the literature would support stapled hemorrhoidopexy as a safe and effect procedure, if performed by inexperienced surgeons, for the wrong indications, or without meticulous attention to operative technique it may be associated with complications. The purpose of the first part of this chapter is to describe a standardized and reproducible technique for stapled hemorrhoidopexy. The second part of the chapter will present possible complications and discuss various "tips and tricks" to avoid their occurrence.

Stapled Hhemorrhoidopexy

Preoperative Preparation

Patient Selection

The PPH operation is suitable for patients with Grade II–IV hemorrhoids and selected patients with symptomatic rectal mucosal prolapse. The patient must be suitable for either general or regional anesthesia. Patients with large external hemorrhoids or skin tags must be aware that these will not be excised as part of the operation but that most reduce in size in the weeks following surgery. Occasionally, troublesome residual skin tags may require surgical excision. Informed consent of the potential risks, benefits, and alternative treatments must be provided.

Patient Preparation

There is some evidence that the perioperative use of lactulose reduces postoperative pain in patients undergoing conventional hemorrhoidectomy. No such data exist concerning its use in stapled hemorrhoidopexy, but logic would suggest that it might also be of some benefit in this situation as well. It is the authors' practice to administer a preoperative rectal enema.

Patient Positioning

The PPH operation may be performed in either the prone jack knife or lithotomy position depending on the surgeon's preference. In the lithotomy position it is important that the hips are fully flexed to expose the entire perineum. This position has the advantage in women of enabling vaginal examination during the operation. This is important to prevent accidental inclusion of the posterior vaginal wall in the staple line. Skin preparation and draping is standard. A gauze swab can usefully be inserted into the lower rectum and withdrawn to show the extent of hemorrhoidal and mucosal prolapse.

Technique for Stapled Hemorrhoidopexy

Circular Anal Dilator Insertion

Four quadrant sutures are inserted at the anal verge, cut long and held with hemostat forceps. Traction on these sutures facilitates insertion of the obturator, which is performed slowly and carefully to avoid iatrogenic internal sphincter trauma (Fig. 6.1a, b). Once the anal canal has been dilated, the obturator is withdrawn and then reinserted covered with the CAD (circular anal dilator). The obturator is withdrawn and the CAD inserted fully into the anal canal. The correct position of the CAD is checked such that the top of the hemorrhoidal columns and the lower rectal mucosa is visible. The stay sutures are then tied to hold the CAD in place (Fig. 6.2a, b)

Placement of the Purse-String Suture

The purse-string suture is next inserted. A 2/0 polypropylene suture on a 30-mm round bodied needle is suitable. Great care must be exercised

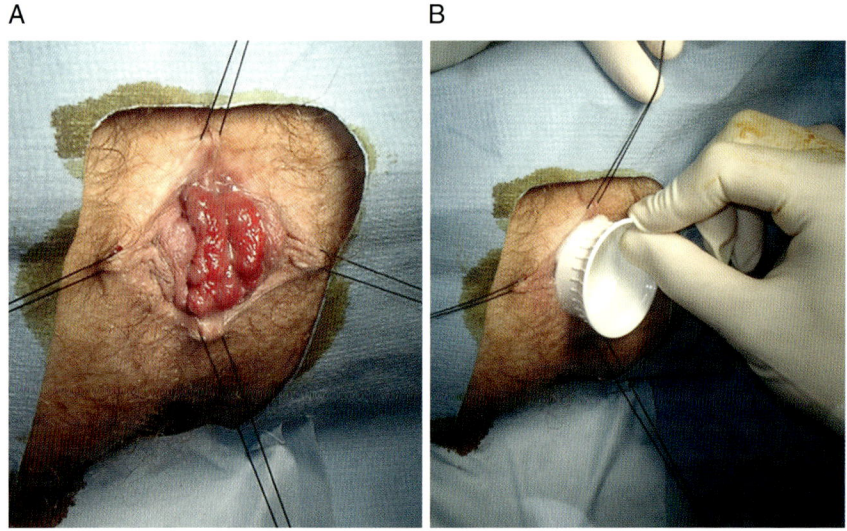

FIG. 6.1. Operative images depicting placement of the stay sutures (**a**) and insertion of the anal dilator (**b**)

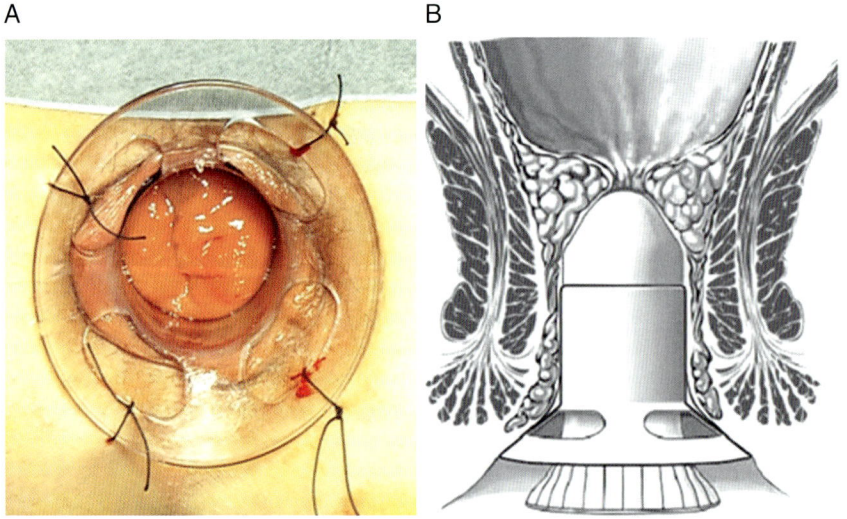

FIG. 6.2. Schematic (**a**) and operative images (**b**) showing correct placement of the CAD into the anal canal

to position the suture correctly at 2 cm above the apex of the hemorrhoidal tissue. The object is not to include the entire hemorrhoidal tissue, but rather a cuff of tissue incorporating normal rectal mucosa and only the apices of the hemorrhoidal pedicles. The suture is submucosal in depth and should not include rectal muscularis propria (Fig. 6.3a, b). The operator must ensure a continuous submucosal purse string avoiding gaps that might later lead to bridges of stapled mucosa. It is important to fully remove the anal retractor and reinsert it in the new position as suturing progresses in a circumferential fashion around the anorectum. This avoids the risk of a spiraling suture line should the anal retractor be rotated within the anorectum. In women, a digital vaginal examination is performed to ensure the purse string has not tethered the posterior vaginal wall. It is important not to pull the purse string closed while checking its position as this may make insertion of the stapler more difficult.

Stapler Insertion

A suitable circular stapling instrument (PPH 33mm, Ethicon Endosurgery) is opened to its full extent and inserted into the anal canal ensuring the head is positioned above the purse string. The purse string is then tied and the ends pulled through the holes in the stapler head using the suture-threading instrument (Fig. 6.4a, b).

Stapler Closure

The suture ends are then be held to apply firm traction on the purse string. The head is closed to its fullest extent by rotating the closure mechanism on the end of the shaft in an anticlockwise direction (Fig. 6.5a, b). It is important to ensure proper alignment of the instrument in the axis of the anal canal. Using the PPH 33mm instrument, closure is confirmed by the presence of the red position marker within the green firing zone on the handle of the instrument. Care is taken in females that the posterior vaginal wall is not included within the head of the instrument.

Firing the Stapler

The stapler is fired by releasing the safety mechanism then closing the handles in a single motion. The purse-string suture is not divided as it is during anterior resection because the suture remains within the instrument head and the ends are within the shaft. Many surgeons prefer to keep the instrument fully closed for 20 s prior to and after firing to maximize clearance of tissue fluid and to encourage staple line hemostasis.

A   B

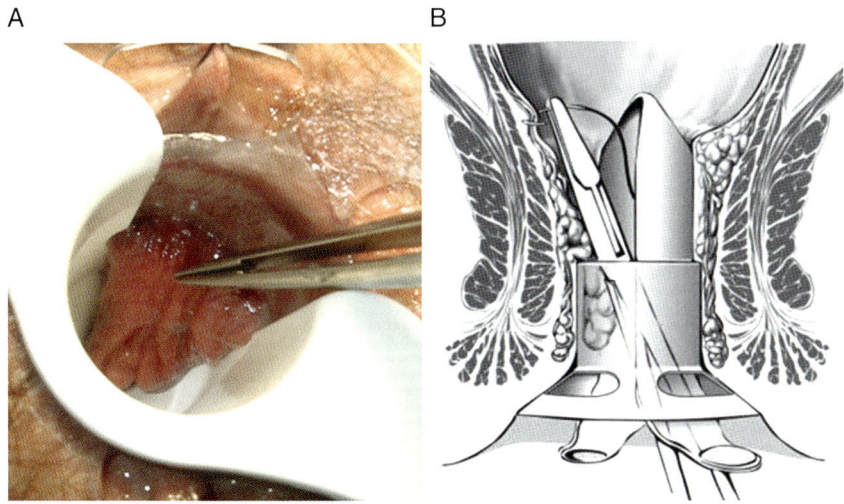

FIG. 6.3. Operative image demonstrating careful identification of the level for purse-string insertion, above the apices of the hemorrhoidal tissue (**a**), and schematic representation of the submucosal placement of the suture

A   B

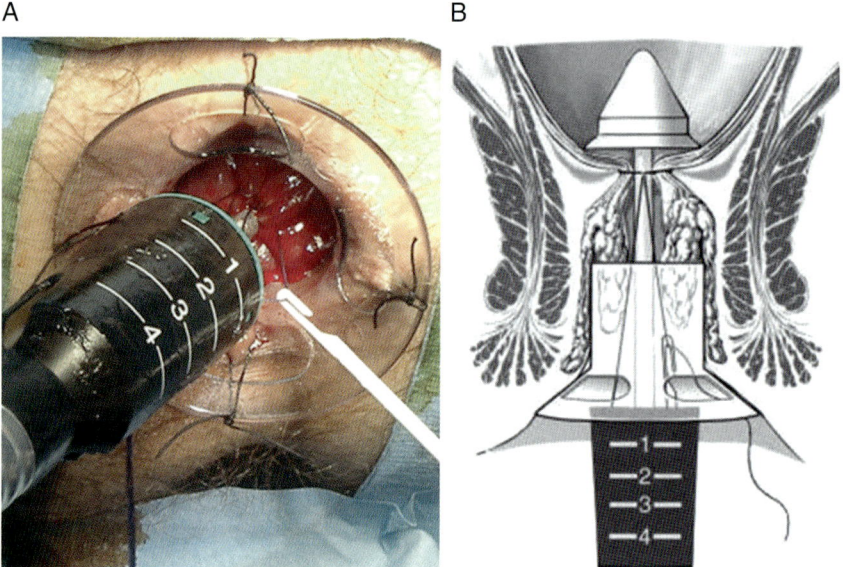

Fig. 6.4. Operative (**a**) and schematic (**b**) images demonstrating the tied purse-string suture which is pulled through the holes in the side of the stapler to provide traction (**a**)

A   B

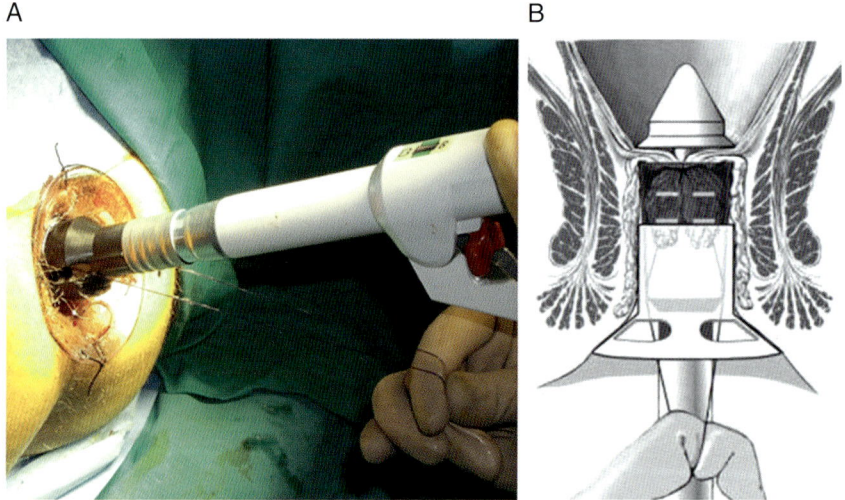

Fig. 6.5. Operative (**a**) and schematic (**b**) images demonstrating traction on the purse-string suture and closure of the stapler with the contained prolapse within the stapler housing

Removing the Stapler

The instrument is removed by opening the head with one half-turn of the closure mechanism in a clockwise direction. A common error is to open the stapler head too widely at this point, which may trap mucosa within the opened instrument head. This makes removal difficult and can damage the anastomosis. The stapler is removed completely, and a gauze swab is inserted into the anal canal to facilitate hemostasis while the excised mucosal doughnut is removed from the

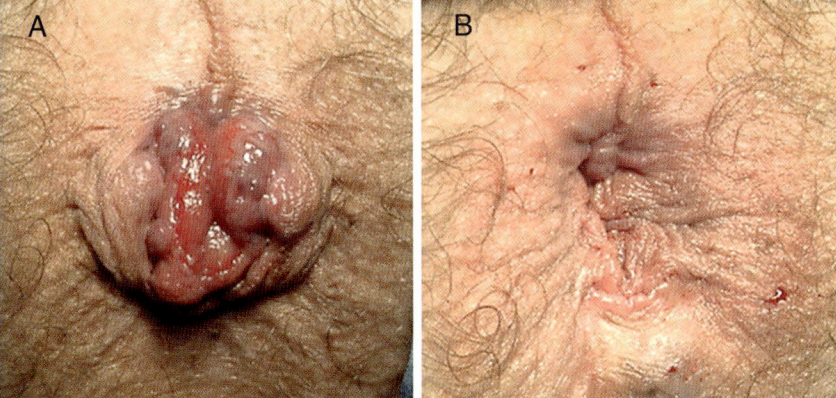

FIG. 6.6   Operative images showing before (**a**) and after (**b**) stapled hemorrhoidopexy

instrument head, examined for adequacy of resection, and sent for histological examination. The CAD should not be removed with the stapling instrument as it is used to facilitate checking of the staple line for bleeding.

Checking the Staple Line

The staple line is checked for bleeding by reinsertion of the anal retractor. Hemostasis is confirmed in each quadrant. Bleeding points should be undersewn using a 3/0 absorbable suture. If necessary, the operation may be completed by insertion of a degradable sponge dressing.

The operative result should be one of complete reduction of hemorrhoidal prolapse with resuspension of the anoderm (Fig. 6.6a, b).

Postoperative Care

Postoperative analgesia in the form of a nonsteroidal anti-inflammatory drug is appropriate (the authors' preference is for Tenoxicam or Diclofenac). Lactulose 10 ml up to three times daily and Metronidazole are continued orally for five days. Patients may be discharged on the evening of, or the day following, operation. Urinary retention is an occasional problem in males, who should be discouraged from drinking excess fluids on the evening of operation. Patients should be warned that passage of small amounts of blood is common in the first few days following operation. Patients should be told to contact their surgeon if there is increasing anorectal pain,

fever, or impaction of feces as these symptoms may indicate perineal infection. Patients should be encouraged to resume normal daily activities as soon as possible.

The Double-PPH Technique

In some rare instances, when dealing with a patient with big mucosal prolapse and hemorrhoids, in order to decrease the chance of prolapse recurrence a variant of the technique has been described: the double-PPH (D-PPH) technique.

The first steps of the D-PPH procedure are the same as those described e. Four quadrant nylon sutures are inserted around the anal verge, cut long and held with hemostat forceps. The obturator is inserted to gently dilate the anal sphincter and then with traction on skin sutures the CAD is fully inserted. Then sutures are tied to hold the CAD in place. The D-PPH technique consists of two symmetrical steps: anterior and posterior prolapse resection. Usually the first step consists of anterior resection: a spatulated retractor is positioned posteriorly to protect the posterior anorectal wall. Then a semicircumferential purse string is placed 2 cm above the top of the hemorrhoidal columns from 9 to 3 o'clock with the patient in lithotomy position. The suture is submucosal in depth and should not include the rectal muscularis propria. To obtain a more symmetrical traction, we perform a second semicircumferential purse string from 9 to 3 o'clock about 2 mm proximal to the first one. At this point the circular stapler (PPH03, Ethicon Endosurgery) is introduced into the anal canal. The purse strings are not tied around the stapler, but the ends are pulled through the side holes in the stapler head. The stapler is fired and resection-anastomosis is performed. The second step consists of a similar resection but is performed in a symmetrical posterior position. This time, a spatulated retractor is positioned anteriorly to protect the anterior anorectal wall from inclusion in the resection. Two semicircumferential purse-string sutures are made from 3 to 9 o'clock, with the second suture at 2 mm proximal to the first. These purse-string sutures start and finish at the ends of the previous anterior staple line. A second PPH03 stapler is inserted into the anal canal and a posterior resection performed. The operation is completed by checking the staple line for hemostasis, and any bleeding points are undersewn using an absorbable suture.

Tips and Tricks

Although stapled hemorrhoidopexy is generally a simple and safe technique, like any other operation there is always a possibility for complications. To minimize the risk of complications, the following tips and tricks may be employed.

Patient Positioning

The procedure can be done either in lithotomy or the prone jack-knife position. If the procedure is to be carried out in lithotomy it is better to place the legs in Allen Stirrups (or an equivalent) with hyperflexion at the hips. This provides better exposure of the perineum and perianal regions and facilitates insertion of the CAD33. The surgeon must not be too close to the surgical field to ensure freedom and ease of movement.

Assessment of Hemorrhoidal Prolapse

To properly assess the extent of hemorrhoidal prolapse it is useful to introduce a dry gauze into the anal canal. By gently extracting the gauze a fecal bolus will be simulated and the extent of the mucosal prolapse will be visible.

Insertion of the Circular Anal Dilator

Preparation and exposure of the surgical field is a basic principle of all operations. In this respect it is essential to take great care not to injure the perineal skin or traumatize the hemorrhoidal tissue before the operation begins.

The first recommendation is to start the procedure by placing stitches at the four cardinal points around the anal canal at a distance of approximately 1 cm from the anal verge. Traction on these four stitches will facilitate the insertion of first the obturator and then the CAD33. The CAD33 should be inserted completely into the anal canal and tightly secured with the anal sutures to prevent inadvertent stapling of the sphincter complex. Some authors recommend the use of a mounted swab to push any tissue trapped between the CAD and the anal canal up into the lower rectum, to ensure complete reduction of prolapsed tissue, although this is not routinely necessary.

Purse-String Placement

With the CAD33 in situ, the dentate line is effaced and not clearly visible. For this reason, it is better to avoid the dentate line as the landmark for positioning of the purse-string suture. Instead, is safer to place the suture 2 cm proximal to the upper end of the hemorrhoidal tissue.

The purse-suture should not be placed too superficial. In addition, the distance between suture bits should be close enough to enable the whole of the circumference of the prolapse to be drawn into the stapler housing when the purse string is tightened.

The anal retractor should never be rotated in the anal canal. Instead, it should be extracted and reinserted as the purse string progresses around the circumference of the anorectum.

PPH03 Insertion, Closure, and Firing

The PPH03 stapler should be introduced completely open and perpendicular to the CAD and anal canal. After its insertion the operator should apply traction to the purse-string suture to ensure that the stapler head is entirely proximal to the prolapsing tissue to be reected. The purse-string suture is then tied tightly around the anvil of the stapler head, but taking care not to snap the suture.

The stapler is closed in two steps. The first step is a graduated closure of the device without applying any traction to the suture ends or any thrust to the stapler. When the graduated scale on the stapler head reaches the position where #2 is level with the anal verge, the second step begins. This involves insertion of the stapler into the anal canal with simultaneous traction applied to the suture ends to draw the prolapsing tissue into the stapler housing. Great care is taken to maintain a 90° angle between the stapler shaft and the CAD such that firing of the stapler results in a resection perpendicular to the anal canal. Waiting 60 s between the complete closure of the stapler and the firing the stapler maximizes compression of tissue fluid from the resection line and enhances hemostasis. At this point the stapler can be fired.

After firing the stapler it is extracted from the CAD by rotating the opening mechanism one half-turn only. The resection specimen and the suture line should always be checked for completeness.

Assessment of the Resection Specimen

The ideal surgical specimen should include a complete submucosal resection, incorporating the lower rectal mucosa and the apices of the hemorrhoidal columns (Fig. 6.7). Occasionally, some smooth muscle fibers may be present which represent the anchoring mechanism of the hemorrhoidal complexes to the underlying internal anal sphincter. Under no circumstances should the resection specimen include squamous mucosa of the anal canal.

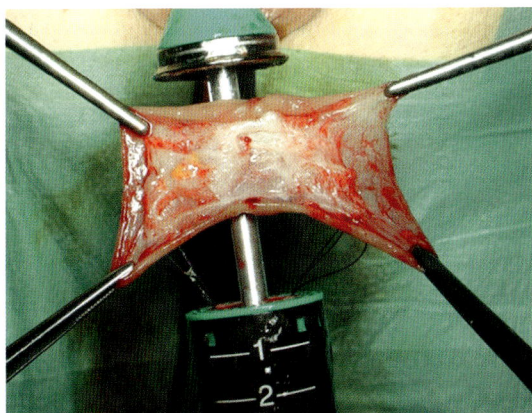

Fig. 6.7. Stapled hemorrhoidopexy resection specimen demonstrating an equally proportioned, circumferential submucosal resection

Checking for Staple Line Bleeding

Homeostasis must be meticulously checked at the staple line. This is particularly so if, as in the majority of cases, the operation is performed as a day-case procedure, when postoperative bleeding will be experience once the patient has been discharged. Excessive bleeding is rare with the PPH03 in comparison to the PPH01 stapler, as the height of the staples has been reduced to increase hemostasis. Should bleeding occur it is recommended to use suction, irrigation, and patience to assure complete hemostasis. Any staple line bleeding point should be controlled with an absorbable 3/0 suture. Diathermy to the staple line should be avoided as it may result in unrecognized thermal spread across the metallic staples with subsequent full-thickness necrosis. Bleeding from the staple line should be distinguished from oozing from residual hemorrhoidal tissue, which is best treated with the use of an absorbable anal dressing, such as Spongostan™. In general, only one or hemostatic sutures are required following the use of the PPH03 stapler.

Some groups recommend leaving a gauze soaked in an oil mixture above of the suture line, and removing it 3 h after the procedure, as an alert to early bleeding complications.

Complications and How to Avoid Them

Stapled hemorrhoidopexy is associated with less postoperative pain and earlier return to normal function when compared to conventional hemorrhoidectomy [1–4]. Although it is a safe procedure, like any other operation, there is always the potential risk of complications (Table 6.1). Similar complications are seen following other interventions for prolapsing hemorrhoids.

Several randomized studies have reported outcomes at short and long-term follow-up, and have failed to demonstrate a significant difference between stapled hemorrhoidopexy and conventional hemorrhoidectomy in terms of fecal incontinence, anal stenosis, persistent pain, and bleeding [5] (see Chap. 8 for further details).

The most common symptoms requiring reintervention are persistent anorectal pain and postoperative bleeding, which may be due to postoperative anal fissure,

TABLE 6.1. Potential complications following stapled hemorrhoidopexy

Early	Late
Bleeding	Recurrent mucohemorrhoidal prolapse
Urinary retention	Fecal incontinence
Fecal impaction	Fecal urgency
Thrombosed external hemorrhoids	Anorectal stricture
Anastomotic dehiscence	Pruritis ani
Anorectal sepsis	Anal discharge
Anal fissure	
Sphincter injury	
Persistent anal pain	
Retrorectal hematoma	
Residual hemorrhoidal prolapse	

recurrent hemorrhoids, or troublesome retained staples [6]. Although a course of conservative treatment (stool softeners, topical anesthetic ointments, ointments to relieve internal sphincter spasm, etc.) may be appropriate, it is unwise to unnecessarily delay reintervention as this may result in a chronicity of symptoms which is difficult to resolve. Most complications can be avoided by good patient selection and a meticulous surgical technique. However, should they occur they are usually amenable to local treatments in the form of rubber band ligation, injection sclerotherapy, lateral internal sphincterotomy, or removal of retained staples. Rarely is further excisional surgery required for residual hemorrhoidal prolapse.

The incidence of complications appears to be related to the learning curve for the procedure [7]. Certainly, the reported incidence of complications shows a large variation, ranging from 6.4 to 31% of cases [8]. Despite this, complications are still been reported by experienced surgeons, but this may be due to extended indications for the procedure or "off-label" use of the stapler.

Following is a compilation of the reported complications encountered following stapled hemorrhoidopexy, together with recommendations on how they can be avoided. For ease of reference they have been classified into "early-" and "late-"occurring complications.

Early Complications

Bleeding

Intraoperative bleeding was relatively common following the use of the PPH01 stapler. Using the more recent PPH03 stapler, significant bleeding is less frequently encountered, with postoperative bleeding rates reduced to 2% as compared to 9% with the PPH01 stapler [9]. Usually, a maximum of 2 hemostatic sutures is required in 80% of cases to control staple line bleeding. When the operation is performed as a day-case procedure, the readmission rate should be less than 3% [10].

Stapled hemorrhoidopexy in fact has a lower incidence of early and late bleeding when compared with conventional hemorrhoidectomy. At 2-weeks follow-up, 67% of patients treated by conventional hemorrhoidectomy complained of persistent bleeding compared with only 20% of patients treated with stapled hemorrhoidopexy. Similarly, at 6-week follow-up the rate of bleeding was significantly reduced following stapled hemorrhoidopexy (0%) compared to conventional hemorrhoidectomy (27%). No difference between the two techniques was demonstrated at 3-month follow-up [11].

In order to minimize postoperative bleeding the following precautions are recommended with the operative technique. After firing the stapler, a careful and thorough examination of the staple line is undertaken. In is regard it may be useful to use irrigation and suction. If any bleeding point is seen, it must be controlled with an absorbable suture and not with the use of cautery, which runs the risk of septic complications should full-thickness necrosis ensue [12]. Other methods to control excessive bleeding include the use of Foley catheter compression or injection of dilute adrenaline into the staple line. The use of an anal tampon has been reported to increase the incidence of postoperative bleeding, due to the trauma sustained during tampon extraction [7].

Urinary Retention

Postoperative urinary retention occurs in approximately 1% of patients treated with stapled hemorrhoidopexy [13], although some authors have reported it in up to 22% of cases [14]. The etiology may be related to postoperative pain and excessive perioperative fluid administration. Restriction of perioperative fluids, the use of local anesthetics at the end of surgery, and attention to adequate postoperative analgesia may help to minimize its incidence. The use of an anal packing may also contribute to urinary retention by exaggerating postoperative pain.

Fecal Impaction

Fecal impaction occurs in < 5% of cases [15]. It must be suspected if the patient reports rectal pressure, constipation, and watery discharge. It can be prevented by attention to a high-fiber diet and the use of stool softeners/laxatives before and after the procedure. A high-fiber diet with the addition of a bulking agent, such as Fybogel™, for 7–14 days is usually enough to prevent its occurrence. The incidence of fecal impaction has been reduced from 7 to 1% after adopting a strategy of routine postoperative lactulose administration [7].

External Hemorrhoidal Thrombosis

Postoperative thrombosis of the external hemorrhoidal plexus occurs in 0.5–6% of cases [16]. It probably results from stasis in the external hemorrhoidal sinusoids secondary to interruption of the superior venous drainage and trauma to the residual nonresected hemorrhoidal tissue. Preventing postoperative constipation may decrease the incidence of this annoying condition.

Anastomotic Dehiscence

The potential for anastomotic dehiscence can be reduced by careful attention to stapler firing. It is recommended to allow 20s following closure of the stapler and its firing, to maximize compression of tissue fluid from the resection line. Similarly, a further 20s should be allowed following firing of the stapler and its removal to overcome the inherent staple memory and to ensure correct closed staple configuration.

It has been suggested that there is a subgroup of patients with fourth-degree hemorrhoids who are at especial risk for anastomotic dehiscence. These patients had hemorrhoidal prolapse which could not be reduced under anesthesia. Adopting a policy of stapled hemorrhoidopexy only for patients with reducible fourth-degree hemorrhoids dramatically decreased the incidence of anastomotic dehiscence after this policy has been observed by their group [16].

Anorectal Sepsis

Serious septic complications have not been observed in published series, except in a German study of 4,635 stapled hemorrhoidopexies where three cases of rectal perforation required treatment with colostomy [17]. However, there have been case reports of retroperitoneal sepsis or Fournier's gangrene after stapled hemorrhoidopexy [8, 12, 19, 20]. These septic complications have also been reported following other procedures for treating hemorrhoids, including injection sclerotherapy [21], rubber band ligation [22], and conventional hemorrhoidectomy either by the Milligan–Morgan or Ferguson technique.

The cause of this polymicrobial infection following stapled hemorrhoidopexy is probably multifactorial. Some argue that including muscle into the stapler increases the risk of this complication. Others suggest that the use of electrocautery on the staple line as a method of hemostasis can result in local full-thickness tissue necrosis with translocation of bacteria into the perirectal tissues [12]. Although there is little evidence to suggest that the routine use of prophylactic antibiotics, mechanical bowel preparation, or rectal enemas reduces the incidence of septic complications, it seems logical to use such strategies as the consequences of perianal/perirectal sepsis should it occur can be quite devastating. The risk of severe perirectal sepsis will also be reduced by avoiding perirectal hematoma formation. This requires the avoidance of muscle incorporation into the anastomosis and attention to hemostasis.

Patients who complain of fever, abdominal pain, urinary retention, or excessive anorectal pain in the postoperative period must be reviewed by a senior surgeon, and if there is any suspicion of impending sepsis an aggressive approach to an early diagnosis and treatment must be taken.

Anal Fissure

Anal fissure has been reported in 0–2.5% of cases following stapled hemorrhoidopexy [23]. It may result from stretching of the anal canal during the insertion of the anal dilator. Using a gentle and progressive digital dilatation of the anal canal before introducing the obturator and CAD33 should decrease the incidence of this painful condition to almost a zero. It will also reduce the risk of iatrogenic sphincter injury.

Sphincter Injury

There has been much concern regarding the reporting of muscle fibers in the resection specimen following stapled hemorrhoidopexy which may be indicative of injury to the underlying internal sphincter. In addition, and the use of a stapling device with a 33-mm anal dilator might result in damage to both internal and external sphincters due to an excessive stretching. Some studies have attempted to assess the degree of sphincter injury by endoanal ultrasound, following both stapled hemorrhoidopexy and conventional hemorrhoidectomy, and have not found any difference between the two techniques [24, 25]. Similarly stapled hemorrhoidopexy has been undertaken with and without the use of the anal dilator. Although avoiding of the anal dilator resulted in fewer sphincter injuries on endoanal ultrasound, there was no difference in continence scores or anal canal pressures [25].

Particular care must be taken in older patients or those with a history of previous anal surgery. Both these groups may have poor rectal reservoir capacity, previous sphincter dysfunction, or impairment of other compensatory mechanisms of continence. In such patients, a standard anoscope, such as an Eisenhammer retractor, may be the preferred method of exposure of the anorectum rather than the PPH anal dilator/CAD33.

Persistent Anal Pain

A low staple line, at or below the anorectal ring, may result in persistent anal pain or bleeding. Some argue that a deep resection with the inclusion of muscle within the anastomosis may precipitate spasm of the puborectalis muscle and result in severe pain [8].

Utmost care must be taken to ensure that the purse-string suture is placed in exactly the correct position, which is 1–2 cm proximal to the uppermost part of the hemorrhoidal pedicles (3–4 cm proximal above the dentate line).

Protracted pain can also be caused by a narrow anal canal, staple line dehiscence, mucosal injury, increased sphincter tone, or anal spasticity [26].

Any unexpected or unexplained anorectal pain following stapled hemorrhoidopexy should be investigated in the first instance by examination under anesthesia to exclude occult injury or septic complications.

Other Complications

Jongen et al. have reported the presence of submucosal cysts at the staple line on endoanal ultrasound examination in 4 out of 654 patients following stapled hemorrhoidopexy [7]. Two of the four patients complained of difficulties in defecation and were treated by resection of the cysts.

There have been two reports of neoplasia in the resection specimen following stapled hemorrhoidopexy [27, 28]. These patients had been reoperated for persistent bleeding. This reinforces the recommendation to subject all resection specimens to histological analysis as neoplastic changes may not be visible to the naked eye.

Late Complications

Recurrent Hemorrhoidal Prolapse

The National Institute for Health and Clinical Excellence (NICE) in the UK published its updated guidance on stapled hemorrhoidopexy in 2007 [29]. This was primarily based on a meta-analysis of 27 randomized clinical trials involving 2,279 patients who underwent either stapled hemorrhoidopexy or conventional hemorrhoidectomy. The results have confirmed previous suggestions that the rate of recurrent prolapse symptoms is greater after the stapling technique [30]. Overall, the rate of recurrent prolapse in the NICE analysis was 5.18 times greater than conventional hemorrhoidectomy ($p = 0.003$). When recurrent prolapse was analyzed at short-term (< 12 months postoperative) and long-term (> 12 months postoperative) follow-up there was an increased rate at each time point, but this only achieved statistical significance for on long-term follow-up.

The results of the NICE analysis are fairly compelling and have caused speculation as to the cause of the increased symptomatic prolapse seen following stapled hemorrhoidopexy. Some authors point to the fact that analysis of recurrent prolapse is often based on patient reported symptoms, and when patients are examined by a clinician the reported prolapse is in fact due to troublesome anal skin tags in over 50% of cases [31]. Although most anal skin tags are small and relatively insignificant, in a few instances when they are large they may cause symptoms due to poor cosmesis or difficulties in perianal hygiene. In such circumstances it is appropriate to offer the patient skin tag excision. If this is envisaged as a potential problem prior to stapled hemorrhoidopexy, then it is wise to counsel the patient that skin tag excision may be necessary at the time of hemorrhoidopexy and that this might add to the degree of postoperative discomfort.

A further question arises as to whether the report increase in recurrent prolapse is due to true recurrence or due to inadequate excision of large volume hemorrhoidal prolapse at the original hemorrhoidopexy, i.e., due to residual hemorrhoidal tissue. The reporting of increased short-term prolapse would suggest that at least an element of the recurrence is actually due to inadequate excision. This is supported by the higher rate of symptomatic prolapse in grade IV hemorrhoidal disease. It is suggested that in large volume grade IV disease the housing of the PPH03 stapler gun is too small to accommodate sufficient prolapse leading to inadequate debulking and a propensity for recurrent symptoms. However, the significant recurrent prolapse found on long-term follow-up also suggests that there may also be an element of de novo hemorrhoidal prolapse.

Thus, when confronted with large volume grade IV hemorrhoidal disease one should give consideration to performing a conventional hemorrhoidectomy rather than the stapling procedure, unless the operator is sufficiently skilled in the double-stapling techniques for anorectal prolapse.

Fecal Incontinence

Anal sphincter anatomy as assessed by endoanal ultrasound has been reported in two series following stapled hemorrhoidopexy [24, 25]. No difference in the incidence of sphincter injury was found when compared with conventional hemorrhoidectomy (conventional hemorrhoidectomy 6.4% vs. stapled hemorrhoidopexy 4%).

Anorectal manometry has been also used to assess sphincter function post stapled hemorrhoidopexy along with patient reported continence scores. No difference between stapled hemorrhoidopexy and conventional hemorrhoidectomy was observed [30].

To avoid problems with postoperative fecal incontinence, it is necessary to identify those patients with potential sphincter dysfunction at the preoperative stage. This can be really achieved by a careful history. One should be wary of women with a complicated obstetric history and patients who have undergone previous anorectal surgery. If there is any suggestion of preoperative sphincter dysfunction either on clinical history or digital rectal examination, then it is mandatory to subject the patient to formal anorectal physiology testing and anorectal ultrasound examination. If sphincter injury or dysfunction is confirmed, then stapled hemorrhoidopexy is probably best avoided.

Other strategies to avoid inadvertent sphincter injury have previously been mentioned, and include the use of gentle digital anal dilatation prior to insertion of the CAD33 anal retractor, and the avoidance of full-thickness resection which might incorporate smooth muscle fibers of the internal sphincter. It is also of importance to avoid placing the purse string and hence the stapled anastomosis too near to the dentate line. If this occurs, it is likely that there will be excessive resection of the transitional epithelium which is important in the rectoanal inhibitory reflex and anal sampling and are integral to normal continence. Staples placed on or near to the dentate line will also put the patient at risk of urgency, which in itself may contribute to fecal incontinence.

Fecal Urgency

Fecal urgency following stapled hemorrhoidopexy has a reported incidence of 2% [32], and this does not differ from that reported following conventional hemorrhoidectomy. Although a single report of fecal urgency affecting 33% of patients has been reported, this does not reflect the general feeling of those regularly performing the procedure [33]. A degree of fecal urgency in the early postoperative period following stapled hemorrhoidopexy may be the result of anal dilatation during the course of the operation. This can usually be expected to resolve with time as normal sphincter function returns. Again, the importance of gentle anal dilatation prior to insertion of the CAD33 anal retractor cannot be overstated.

Anorectal Stricture

Reported rates of anal stenosis/stricture following stapled hemorrhoidopexy range from 0 to 10% [34]. Most of the cases are actually mild and due to stricturing at the stapled anastomosis rather than the true anal stenosis seen after conventional hemorrhoidectomy. Anastomotic strictures can be readily dealt with by gentle digital dilatation in the outpatient clinic, provided they are appreciated at an early stage when the stricture is still "soft" rather than fibrotic. For this reason it is generally recommended that patients are seen at 3–4 weeks following stapled hemorrhoidopexy when a digital rectal examination should be performed. If follow-up examination is delayed to 6 weeks or later then any stricture is likely to be fibrotic and in such circumstances will require four quadrant stricturoplasty under general anesthesia.

Pruritis

Pruritis may be due to large anal skin tags or to a previous or new mild incontinence with anal seepage. In the absence of skin tags or anal seepage, others causes must be ruled out (infectious, eczema, psoriasis, etc.) and treated appropriately. If residual anal skin tags are symptomatic and causing problems with personal hygiene and pruritis, then simple excision under general anesthetic is recommended. Anal discharge when analyzed in a meta-analysis of 275 patients was found to be more common after conventional hemorrhoidectomy as compared to the stapling technique [35].

Summary

Reasonable evidence is now available to support the claim that stapled hemorrhoidopexy is a safe and effective technique for the treatment of prolapsing symptomatic hemorrhoids. However, like any other surgical procedure, if performed by inexperienced surgeons, on the wrong patients, or without due care to surgical technique, complications may result. A standardized technique for stapled hemorrhoidopexy has been presented which should minimize adverse events. Postoperative complications are no more frequent following stapled hemorrhoidopexy as compared to conventional hemorrhoidectomy. The reported complications following stapled hemorrhoidopexy have been discussed along with tips and tricks to avoid their occurrence. It remains that the best way to minimize complications is through the excellent training of surgeons, appropriate patient selection, and meticulous technique.

References

1. Rowsell M, Bello M, Hemingway DM. Circumferential mucosectomy (stapled hemorrhoidectomy) versus conventional haemorrhoidectomy: randomized controlled trial. Lancet 2000; 355: 768–769
2. Mehigan BJ, Monson JR, Hartley JE. Stapling procedure for hemorrhoids versus Milligan-Morgan haemorrhoidectomy: randomized controlled trial. Lancet 2000; 355: 782–785
3. Boccasanta P, Capretti PG, Venturi M, et al. Randomised controlled trial between stapled circumferential mucosectomy and conventional circular haemorrhoidectomy in advanced haemorrhoids with external mucosal prolapse. Am J Surg 2001; 182: 64–68
4. Ho YH, Cheong WK, Tsang C, et al. Stapled haemorrhoidectomy cost and effectiveness. Randomized, controlled trial including incontinence scoring, anorectal manometry, and endoanal ultrasound assessments at up to three months. Dis Colon Rect 2000; 43: 1666–1675
5. Ganio E, Altomare DF, Milito G, et al. Long term outcome of a multicentre randomized clinical trial of stapled haemorrhoidopexy versus Milligan Morgan haemorrhoidectomy. Br J Surg 2007; 94: 1033–1037
6. Brusciano L, Ayabaca M, Pescatori M, et al. Reinterventions after complicated or failed stapled hemorrhoidectomy. Dis Colon Rectum 2004; 47: 1846–1851
7. Jongen J, Bock JU, Peleikis HG, et al. Complications and reoperations in stapled anopexy: learning by doing. Int J Colorectal Dis 2006; 21: 166–171
8. Ravo B, Amato A, Bianco V, et al. Complications after stapled haemorrhoidectomy: can they be prevented? Tech Coloproctol 2002; 6: 83–88
9. Angelone G, Giardello C, Prota C. Bleeding after stapled haemorrhoidopexy using the new PPH 03 stapler device. Experience and results in 100 consecutive patients. Chir Ital 2007; 59: 225–229

10. Beattie GC, McAdam TK, McIntosh SA, et al. Day case stapled haemorrhoidopexy for prolapsing piles. Colorectal Dis. 2006; 8: 56–61

11. Racalbuto A, Aliotta I, Corsaro G, et al. Hemorrhoidal stapled prolapsectomy vs Milligan-Morgan hemorrhoidectomy: a long term randomized trial. Int J Colorectal Dis 2001; 19: 239–44

12. Maw A, Eu KW, Seow-Choen F. Retroperitoneal sepsis complicating stapled hemorrhoidectomy: report of a case and review of the literature. Dis Colon Rect 2002; 45: 826–828

13. Oughriss M, Yver R, Faucheron JL. Complications of stapled hemorrhoidectomy: a French multicentric study. Gastroenterol Clin Biol 2005; 29: 429–433

14. Ortiz H, Marzo J, Armendariz P. Randomized clinical trial of stapled hemorrhoidopexy versus conventional diathermy haemorrhoidectomy. Br J Surg 2002; 89: 1376–1381

15. Plocek MD, Kondylis LA, Duhan-Floyd N, et al. Hemorrhoidopexy staple line height predicts return to work. Dis Colon Rectum 2006; 49: 1905–1909

16. Shalaby R, Desoky A. Randomized clinical trial of stapled versus Milligan Morgan haemorrhoidectomy. Br J Surg 2001; 88: 1049–1053

17. Herold A, Kirsch JJ. Pain after stapled hemorrhoidctomy. Lancet 2000; 356: 2187

18. Molloy RG, Kingmore D. Life threatening pelvic sepsis after stapled haemorrhoidectomy. Lancet 2000; 355: 810

19. Ripetti V, Caricato M, Arullani A. Rectal perforation, retropneumoperitoneum and pneumomediastinum after stapling procedure for prolapsed hemorrhoids: report of a case and subsequent considerations. Dis Colon Rectum 2002; 45: 268–270

20. Bonner C, Prohm P, Storkel S. Fournier gangrene as a rare complication after stapled haemorrhoidectomy. Case report and review of the literature. Chirurg 2001; 72: 1464–1470

21. Barwell J, Watkins RM, Lloyd Davies E, Wilkins DC. Life threatening retroperitoneal sepsis after haemorrhoidal injection sclerotherapy: report of a case. Dis Colon Rectum 1999; 42: 421–423

22. O'Hara VS. Fatal clostridial infection following haemorrhoidal banding. Dis Colon Rectum 1980; 23: 570–571

23. Mascagni D, Zeri KP, Di Matteo FM, et al. Stapled heemorrhoidectomy: surgical notes and results. Hepato-gastroenterol 2003, 50: 1878–1882

24. Brown SR, Ballan K, Ho E, et al. Stapled mucosectomy for acute thrombosed circumferentially prolapsed piles: a prospective randomized comparison with conventional haemorrhoidectomy. Colorectal Dis 2001; 3: 175–178

25. Ho YH, Seow Choen F, Tsang C, Eu KW. Randomized trial assessing anal sphincter injuries after stapled haemorrhoidectomy. Br J Surg 2001; 88: 1449–1455

26. Cheetham MJ, Mortensen NJ, Nystrom PO, et al. Persistent pain and faecal urgency after stapled haemorrhoidectomy. Lancet 2000; 356: 826–828

27. Watson AJ, McLaren CM, Chapman AD, et al. Further cautionary tales from histopathology of stapled hemorrhoidopexy specimens. Colorectal Dis 2003, 5: 270–272

28. Ortiz H, Marzo J, Armendariz P. Stapled hemorrhoidectomy vs diathermy excision for fourth degree hemorrhoids: a randomized, clinical trial and review of the literature. Dis Colon Rectum 2005; 48: 809–815

30. Nisar PJ, Acheson AG, Neal KR, Scholefield JH. Stapled haemorrhoidopexy compared with conventional haemorrhoidectomy: systematic review of randomized controlled trials. Dis Colon Rect 2004; 47: 1837–1845

31. Gania E, Altomare DF, Gabrielli F, Milito G, Canuti S. Prospective randomized mulitcentre trial comparing stapled with open haemorrhoidectomy. Br J Surg 2001; 88: 669–764

32. Tjandra J, Chan M. Systematic review on the procedure for prolapse and hemorrhoids (stapled hemorrhoidopexy). Dis Colon Rect 2007; 50: 878–892

33. Thaha MA, Kazmi SA, Irvine LA, et al. New onset fecal urgency and its impact on recovery following circular stapled anopexy: preliminary results of a multicentre randomized controlled trial. Br J Surg 2003; 90: S1

34. Peng BC, Jayne DG, Ho YH. Randomized trial of rubber band ligation vs stapled hemorrhoidectomy for prolapsed piles. Dis Colon Rect 2003; 46: 291–297

35. Lan P, Wu X, Zhou X, et al. The safety and efficacy of stapled hemorrhoidectomy in the treatment of hemorrhoids: a systematic review and meta-analysis of ten randomized control trials. Int J Colorectal Dis 2006; 21: 172–178

Chapter 7
Stapled Transanal Rectal Resection Procedure

D.G. Jayne and A. Stuto

Abstract The original stapled transanal resection (STARR) technique utilized two firings of a PPH01 stapler to achieve separate anterior and posterior resections of the distal rectum. More recently, a device specifically designed for STARR has been introduced: the Contour Transtar. This enables a greater extent of prolapse to be resected as a single specimen. Both techniques are described in detail together with "tips and tricks" for a successful outcome.

Introduction

The experience with stapled prolapsectomy for the treatment of hemorrhoids led to the idea that resection of internal mucosal prolapse could improve rectal evacuation. Based on this idea, and accompanied with evidence gained from cadaveric studies, Antonio Longo proposed the full-thickness resection of the lower rectum to treat obstructed defecation syndrome (ODS) in patients with rectocele and rectal intussusception. The first presentation of this novel technique was made by Longo during a workshop held in Vienna, at the St. Elizabeth Hospital, in December 2000. To this workshop, which was entitled "Stapled Rectocele Repair," six Italian surgeons with the most experience in stapled hemorrhoidopexy were invited. Longo demonstrated his novel technique for repairing rectoceles associated with ODS and explained the rationale. An exciting brainstorming session transpired which culminated in Paolo Boccasanta proposing the acronym stapled transanal rectal resection (STARR) for the new technique.

The Original Technique

The original technique was presented by Longo in Ft. Lauderdale, Florida, in 2003 [1]. The aim of the STARR procedure was to produce a full-thickness rectal resection, and it was distinguished from previous operations for rectal prolapse, such as Altemeir's procedure, by virtue of the fact that external dissection of the rectum was not required, but rather STARR was performed solely by a transanal approach. The resection and the anastomosis are performed in a single step, minimizing the risks of dehiscence and fistula formation. Before going into the details of the original technique it is important to underline that at the time STARR was proposed there was no dedicated stapling device available to perform it. Instead, the PPH-01 kit and its technique of application were modified to produce a full-thickness resection. The PPH01 device, used for both stapled hemorrhoidopexy and STARR, is a circular stapler capable of producing a 360° rectal resection in a single firing. However, unlike stapled hemorrhoidopexy, two staplers are required for STARR in order to resect the rectal intussusception anteriorly (incorporating any rectocele) and posteriorly. The use of a single stapler is insufficient to resect the necessary amount of prolapse found in ODS.

D. Jayne and A. Stuto (eds.), *Transanal Stapling Techniques for Anorectal Prolapse*,
DOI: 10.1007/978-1-84800-905-9_7, © Springer-Verlag London Limited 2009

The operation is performed under general or caudal anesthesia, with the patient in a "forced" lithotomy position (i.e., with the hips flexed greater than 90°). This helps to expose the perineum and provides the best operative view for the surgeon.

The circular stapler with a disposable circular anal dilator a and anoscope is used (PPH-01™; Ethicon Endo-Surgery, Inc.). The first step of the procedure is similar to the PPH technique and consists of preparing the operative field with full insertion of the anal dilator. In order to do this, the anal verge is gently dilated with an Eisenhammer retractor which also facilitates operative evaluation of the anatomy and the extent of distal rectal prolapse.

Four radial stitches are inserted into the perianal skin at the distance of 1 cm from the anal verge to better expose and evert the anal canal. The lubricated obturator is gently introduced and left in place for 30–60 s, following which the lubricated anal dilator (CAD) is introduced into the anal canal. Traction on the stay sutures aids insertion of the CAD by applying countertraction. Once fully inserted, the CAD is secured in place by tying the stay sutures. We strongly believe that the CAD must be securely fixed to the skin by the suture and not held by an assistant's hand. Moreover, the CAD should be removed only at the very end of the procedure.

After the CAD has been positioned and secured, a malleable retractor (spatula) is passed through the posterior window of the CAD and inserted 4–5 cm into the anorectum. This retractor is used to protect the posterior rectal wall and exclude it during resection of the anterior rectal wall.

In order to perform the resection and anastomosis, the desired amount of prolapse must be captured and brought into the housing of the PPH device. This has to be carefully judged by the operating surgeon.

The anoscope (PSA 33) is inserted into the CAD and three separate one-half (180°) purse-string sutures, incorporating mucosa, submucosa, and rectal muscle wall, are placed. The first suture is placed 2 cm above the hemorrhoidal apices or at least 2 cm. above the anorectal ring. This suture position should incorporate the distal extent of rectocele and internal rectal prolapse. We recommend the use of a 2/0 monofilament suture on a 26-mm rounded body needle for this purpose. The first suture is placed starting at 9 o'clock and moving counterclockwise to reach 3 o'clock position. The next hemipurse-string suture is positioned 1 cm cranial to the first and placed in the same manner. A third suture is then placed 1 cm cranial to the second. The distance between the first and the last suture should be approximately 2 cm. Gentle traction on the three sutures will reveal the extent of the prolapse to be resected (Fig. 7.1). During placement of the anterior purse-string sutures care must be taken not to include the vaginal wall. For this reason, it is recommended that the vagina is check both visually and by digitation after each purse-string suture is placed.

Once the anterior purse-string sutures are in place, the anterior resection can be undertaken. A malleable retractor is inserted into the lower window of the CAD and guided 4–5 cm into the distal rectum to protect the posterior rectal wall during the anterior resection (Fig. 7.1). The PPH 33-mm circular stapler is fully opened and the head placed above the three anterior hemipurse-string sutures. The sutures are left free and threaded through the openings in either side of the stapler housing. Before firing the stapler a vaginal retractor (e.g., Simms retractor) is positioned to lift the

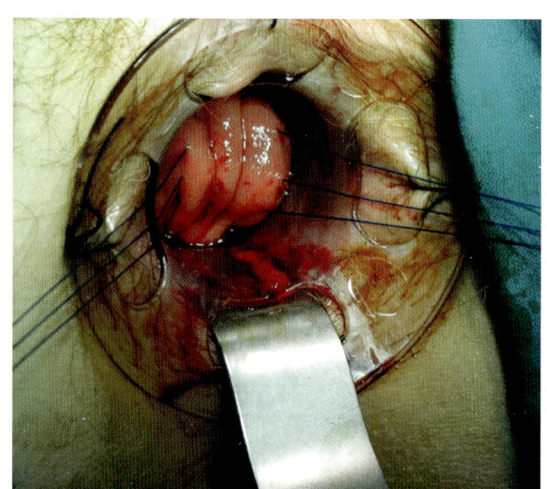

FIG. 7.1. STARR PPH01 technique: the three anterior hemipurse-string sutures have been placed approximately 1 cm apart from the 9 o'clock to 3 o'clock positions. Traction on the sutures reveals the extent of the prolapse to be resected. The posterior rectal wall is protected by a malleable retractor inserted through the lower window in the CAD

uterus and posterior vagina floor and prevent its entrapment in the stapler jaws. The vaginal floor must be carefully checked by digital examination during closure of the stapler: it should slide easily over the stapler head. During closure of the stapler the purse-string sutures are used to apply traction toward the surgeons, while at the same time the stapler is gently advanced into the anorectum (Fig. 7.2). This maneuver will help capture the prolapsing tissue into the stapler housing. The stapler is fully closed such that the red indicator on the stapler shaft reaches the end of the green scale, and fired. The stapler is withdrawn by twisting the opening mechanism by one-half turn and gently withdrawing.

The procedure is now repeated for the posterior rectal wall, with the malleable retractor inserted into the upper window of the CAD. Three separated one-half (180°) purse-string sutures are inserted above the hemorrhoid apices, including mucosa, submucosa, and rectal wall. These posterior hemipurse-string sutures are placed starting at 3 o'clock, where one end of the anterior anastomosis is visible, and finish at 9 o'clock where the other end of the anterior anastomosis is found. The second stapler device is inserted fully opened, then closed, fired, and withdrawn. A small mucosal bridge with a staple connecting the two edges of the anastomosis is frequently encountered and must be divided with scissors (Fig. 7.3a, b).

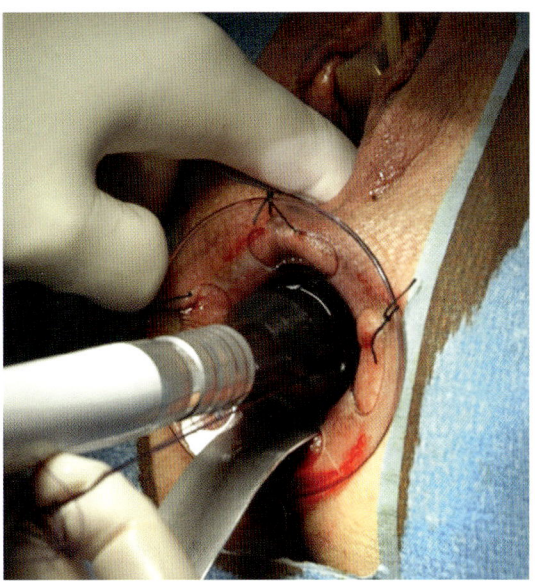

FIG. 7.2. STARR PPH01 technique: the traction sutures are threaded through the side holes in the PPH01 stapler which is inserted into the anorectum. The stapler is closed while maintaining traction on the sutures and checking the vagina to ensure that the vaginal mucosa has not been inadvertently included between the stapler jaws

The combined effect of the anterior and posterior resections is a full-thickness circumferential rectal resection. The final step is to check for bleeding from the suture line, paying particular attention

A   B

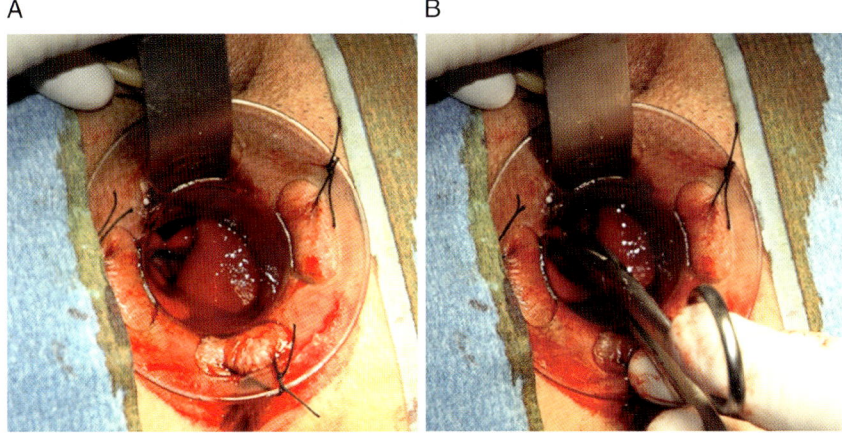

FIG. 7.3. STARR PPH01 technique: A small mucosal bridge is frequently encountered following the anterior and posterior resection (**a**), and must be divided with scissors (**b**)

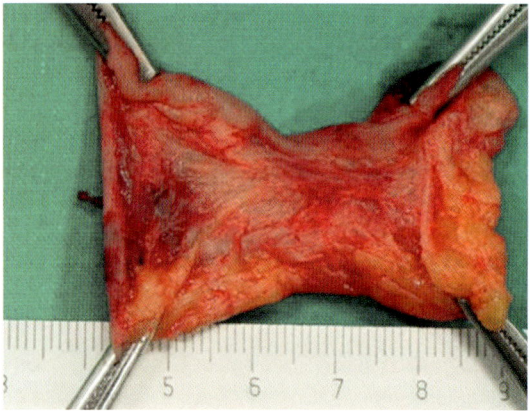

Fig. 7.4. Anterior resection specimen showing full-thickness resection

to the so called lateral dog ears. The "dog ears" represent the crossing of two anterior and posterior stapled anastomosis at the 3 and 9 o'clock positions. Resorbable 3/0 sutures are recommended to secure hemostasis.

The specimen is checked to determine adequacy of resection, both in resection height and inclusion of the full rectal wall thickness Fig. 7.4.

At this stage the CAD can be removed and if desired a gauze swab can be placed above the stapled anastomosis to warn of postoperative bleeding; it is removed approximately 3 h later if no bleeding has ensued.

The patients should receive a short course of antibiotics, and for this purpose a cephalosporin together with metronidazole is recommended at induction of anesthesia. Postoperative antibiotics are not usually necessary.

Tips and Tricks

The best advice for ensuring good results from STARR, or any other surgical procedure, is to correctly identify those patients most suitable for the procedure. This topic is covered elsewhere (Chap. 5).

Although the procedure can be performed in a relatively short space of time (on average 45 min), it is vital that a meticulous technique is employed and attention to detail in each step of the procedure is necessary.

The patient's position on the operating table must be in forced lithotomy to ensure adequate exposure of the perineum. It is not recommended to attempt STARR in the prone jacknife position as this limits access to the vagina, which is necessary to ensure that it is not inadvertently included in the staple line.

During placement of the hemipurse-string sutures, the stitch depth should not be too superficial, but neither should it be placed as deep as possible; the aim is to catch all layers of the rectal wall. Full-thickness rectal resection does not depend on the depth of the needle bite, but on the traction placed on the purse strings during the closure and firing of the stapler.

The use of a vaginal retractor during closure of the stapler is recommended to elevate the uterus and flatten the posterior vaginal wall. This will facilitate digital examination of the vagina. Lifting the uterus will have the added benefit of closing the pouch of Douglas and minimizing the risk of small bowel (enterocele) sliding into the pouch and inadvertent injury.

After closing the stapler it is recommended that the operator waits for at least 20 s before firing: the resulting compression will help to eliminate tissue fluid and produce a better resection and more secure anastomosis. In the same fashion, it is recommended to wait a further 20 s between firing the stapler and its opening and removal, which allows the titanium staples to lose their inherent metallic memory.

During the posterior resection it is important to place the hemipurse-string sutures at least 2 cm. from the hemorrhoidal apices (anorectal ring). This avoids the anastomosis being too low and impinging on the sensitive anoderm with resulting excessive postoperative pain.

Complications and How to Avoid Them

Bleeding. Postoperative bleeding requiring prolonged hospital stay and/or reintervention occurs in 2–5% of cases [2]. The only tip to avoid this is a meticulous checking for bleeding from the anastomotic line after firing the stapler. The most commonly encountered site of bleeding is at the so called dog ears. It is therefore recommended to insert two hemostatic stitches in this area, one on each side, even if there is no significant bleeding.

Urgency. Postoperative fecal urgency is a common symptom in the first few weeks after STARR. In around 70–80% of the patients it is self-limiting and resolves within one month after surgery. In the remaining patients urgency can last for more than 3 months. The explanation for post-STARR urgency is not clear; therefore, there are no obvious tips or tricks to follow during the procedure to avoid its occurrence. Personal experience suggests that one of the causes of urgency might be a low staple line, especially on the posterior aspect. An alternative explanation for urgency might be due to inadequate prolapse resection: it has been observed that fewer patients appear to complain of fecal urgency following the newer Contour Transtar procedure, although this impression has not been confirmed.

Enterocele/Sigmoidocele. STARR is contraindicated when internal rectal prolapse coexists with a fixed enterocele, i.e., an enterocele which is present even at rest and not just on straining to defecate. However, STARR can be performed if an enterocele/sigmoidocele is dynamic and occurs only on straining. In such circumstances, additional care should be exercised to ensure that the patient is in sufficient Trendelenburg position (head-down), and a retractor is used to lift up the uterus. An alternative strategy is to insert a laparoscope to retract any small bowel/colon from the pelvis and to perform the STARR under laparoscopic vision.

Retained staples. In the case where symptoms of urgency, pain, bleeding, or mucous discharge persist for more than 3 months after surgery, the anastomotic line should be inspected for the presence of retained staples. This is best done under anesthesia when any retained staples can be removed and a further inspection undertaken for anastomotic strictures or other causes of symptoms. Usually, anastomotic strictures are readily amenable to radial stricturoplasty and dilatation.

Variations on the Original Technique

The most important variation of the original STARR technique, as it was first proposed by Longo in 2000, has been the method for capturing the rectal prolapse within the stapler. Instead of using the original three hemipurse-string sutures to retract the anterior and posterior prolapse, the rectal wall can be retracted using three short running sutures as shown in Fig. 7.5a, b. These sutures are placed at 10-, 12-, and 2-o'clock anteriorly and at 4-, 6-, and 8-o'clock posteriorly.

A   B

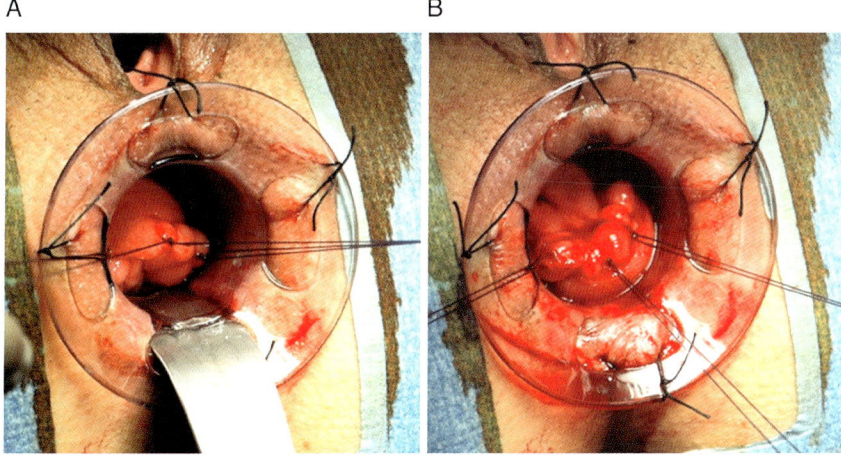

FIG. 7.5. STARR PPH01-modified technique (**a**) 3 sutures are placed at the 10-, 12-, and 2 o'clock positions. The two ends of the 12 o'clock suture are split and separately combined with the 10- and 2 o'clock sutures to give a uniform traction on the anterior rectal prolapse; (**b**) in similar fashion three sutures are used to provide traction on the posterior rectal prolapse

Prolapsing the rectal wall in this way results in a bigger resection and better visualization.

The Contour Transtar Device: STARR with Transtar

Experience with the STARR technique, as proposed by Antonio Longo [1], has proved it to be highly beneficial in the treatment of obstructed defecation symptoms in patients with intussusception and rectocele [2–8]. But the original technique was performed with the PPH01 stapler, which was not designed for this purpose. The PPH01 was created for submucosal hemorrhoidal resection. One of the criticisms of the STARR performed with two PPH01 staplers was that the resection could not be performed equally around the circumference of the rectal wall due to the fact that two separate anterior and posterior stapler firings were required. This inevitably resulted in lateral "dog ears" where full-thickness resection was deficient. In addition, the resection was performed in a "blind" manner and with the volume of resection being determined by the capacity of the stapler housing rather than by the size of the prolapse. In other words, it was not possible to tailor the extent of the resection to the size of the prolapse. Moreover, abuse of the technique left it open to potentially serious complications

[9]. Although the functional results achieved with the PPH01 STARR were good, there was room for improvement in the stapler to give the surgeon a degree of flexibility to improve the anatomical correction necessary for best functional outcome.

For this reason a new stapler was devised specifically for use in STARR: a curved cutting stapler which looked like a Contour40 stapler but with a 30-mm staple line. Ethicon Endo-Surgery (Cincinnati, OH, USA) has marketed this device under the name of Contour Transtar (STR5G). The device is a reloadable and supplied in a kit with an Obturator, a Circular Anal Dilator, and a fenestrated Anoscope (Fig. 7.6).

Surgical Technique

Preoperatively, bowel cleansing and antibiotic prophylaxis is administered, according to local preference. The patient is placed in the lithotomy position under spinal or general anesthesia. Any external prolapse is reduced manually. The anal dilator is gently introduced and fixed to the perianal skin with four retaining sutures.

Step 1: Parachute suture placement. The first suture is placed at the apex of the prolapse, which is best demonstrated by the introduction and withdrawal of a dry swab. Alternatively, the apex of the prolapse can be captured by introducing the

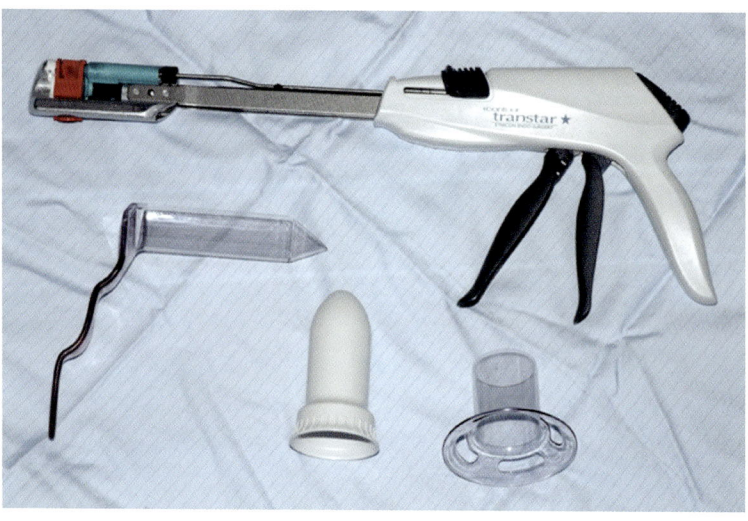

FIG. 7.6. The Contour Transtar kit consisting of stapling gun (STR5G), obturator, circular anal dilator, and fenestrated anoscope

anoscope and applying a suture above the CAD margin; the height of this suture determines the amount of the prolapse to be removed and is usually 2–5 cm from the CAD margin (Fig. 7.7). Three or four full bits of the prolapse are taken, traveling approximately 2–3 cm around the rectal circumference. The suture is then loosely knotted. In a similar fashion, four or five sutures are inserted in a counterclockwise fashion around the entire rectal circumference. Uniform traction on the sutures allows the length of the internal rectum prolapse to be evaluated; this is referred to as the "parachute maneuver" (Fig. 7.8).

Step 2: Longitudinal opening of the prolapse. When the height of the intussusception is >3 cm, one suture (the radial suture) is inserted at the base of the invaginated prolapse at the 3 o'clock position. This suture is knotted tightly to reduce the length of the prolapse. The stapling device is introduced into the rectum with the opened jaws inserted within the loop of the radial suture, making sure it is inserted well inside the rectal lumen, completely surrounded by the prolapsed tissue. During the first cut, the head of the stapler is radial to the Circular Anal Dilator, such that a cut is made perpendicular to the axis of the prolapse, effectively opening up the prolapse (Fig. 7.9). This is facilitated by applying

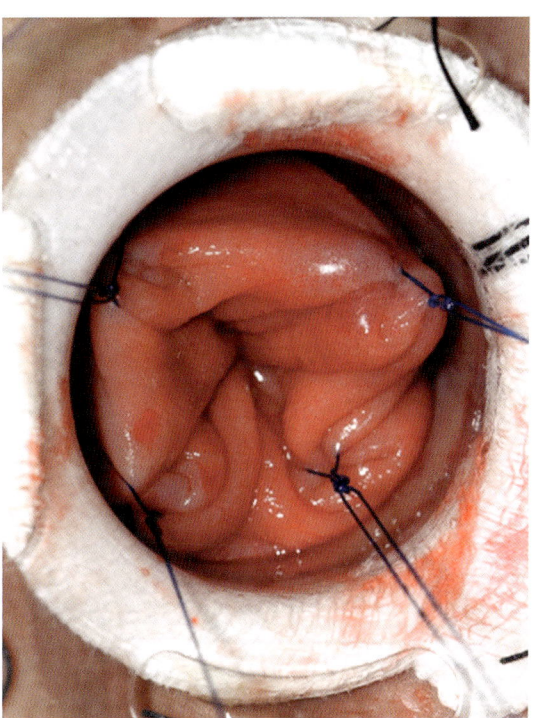

FIG. 7.8. STARR with Contour Transtar: four traction sutures are placed at the 2-, 10-, 8-, and 4 o'clock positions gathering up the prolapse and defining the extent of resection

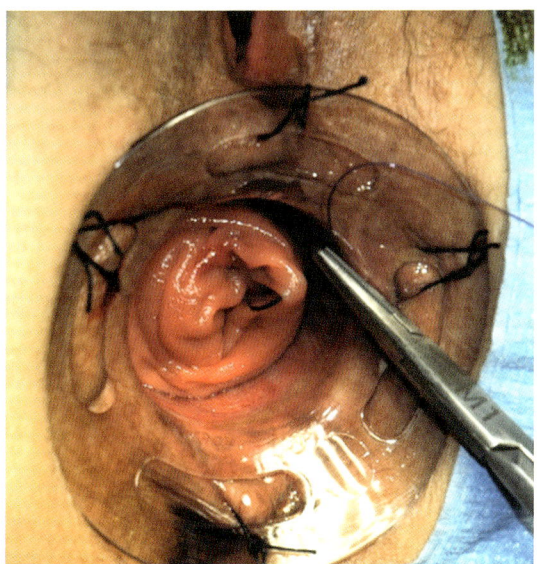

FIG. 7.7. STARR with Contour Transtar: the first suture is placed in the apex of the prolapse at the 2 o'clock position

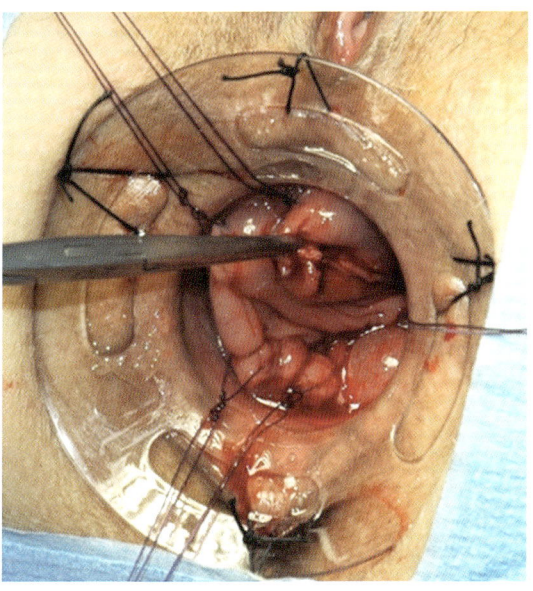

FIG. 7.9. STARR with Contour Transtar: the first cut with the Contour Transtar is made radial to the axis of the rectum, opening up the prolapse and determining the extent of resection

traction to the left on the redial suture, drawing the prolapse into the stapler jaws. This first cut must be made at the 3 o'clock position to minimize the possibility of inadvertent vaginal injury. Once fully inserted, the retaining pin of the stapler is closed manually, checking that the vagina remains free with an examining finger. The device is then closed and fired. The device is removed from the rectum and a hemostatic suture is inserted at the apex of the opened prolapse marking the beginning and end of the circumferential resection and reinforcing the anastomosis. This suture acts as a reference point to guide circumferential resection and helps to avoid spiraling of the anastomosis.

Step 3: Circumferential resection. A clamp is placed on the proximal end of the first cut, thus ensuring the correct depth for the circumferential resection and facilitating manipulation of the prolapse. Applying traction to the "parachute," the device is introduced into the rectum with the opened jaws parallel to the Circular Anal Dilator (CAD) and moved counterclockwise, pulling the prolapse inside the jaws of the device. Again, the vagina is checked with the finger, and a constant and gentle traction is applied to the parachute. The retaining pin is closed manually followed by the stapler, which is then fired. The device is removed, the cartridge replaced, and the procedure repeated sequentially along the rectal circumference (Fig. 7.10). It is important to apply a constant traction on the parachute sutures throughout the procedure to ensure an equal amount of tissue is resected around the circumference, with the resection beginning and ending at the same point in the 3 o'clock position. As a rule, four to six stapler firings are needed on average to complete the resection, but this may vary depending on the amount of prolapse to be resected.

Particular attention must be paid during the anterior part of the resection so as not to inadvertently incorporate extrarectal tissues (vagina, enterocele, sigmoidocele) in the resection. This is helped by digital examination of posterior vaginal wall, the use of vaginal retractors, and a Trendelenburg position. The intersection of sequential staple lines represents a point of potential weakness, and these areas should be carefully inspected at the end of the procedure and additional reinforcing sutures inserted as necessary. Hemostasis is secured with the use of interrupted 3/0 vicryl sutures as required. Cautious removal of the anoscope completes the operation.

A Cautionary Note

Although preliminary results of STARR performed with the Contour Transtar stapler are very encouraging, its safety and efficacy has not been formally evaluated. Feasibility and safety studies are ongoing. At present, it is recommended that the Contour

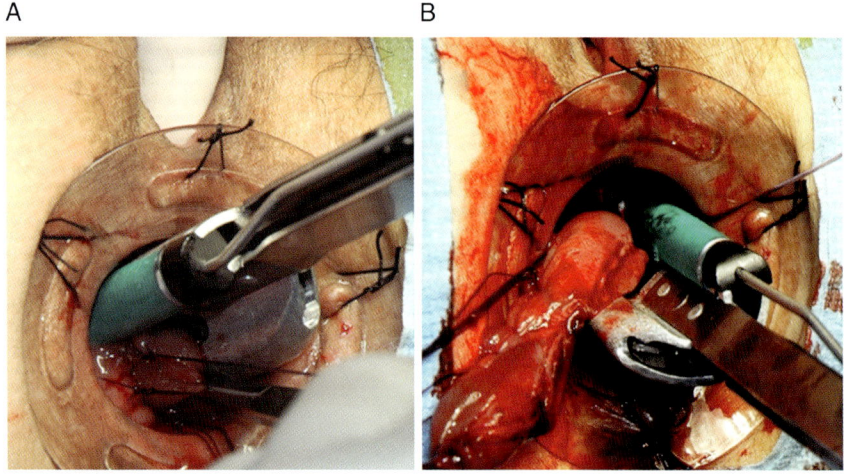

FIG. 7.10. STARR with Contour Transtar: sequential circumferential resection of the prolapse. (**a**) the first cut includes the anterior prolapse and an examining finger is used to ensure the vagina has not been inadvertently incorporated; (**b**) the last cut completes the circumferential resection, beginning and ending at the same point. The resected prolapse emerges from the CAD as a "sausage-" like structure

Transtar stapler should be only used by colorectal surgeons who have been specifically trained in its use and who are competent with other transanal stapling techniques. Any surgeon undertaking this procedure should be aware of the potential complications described earlier and familiar with strategies to avoid them.

References

1. Longo A. Obstructed defecation because of rectal pathologies. Novel surgical treatement: rectal resection (STARR). Proceedings of the 14th Annual International Colo-rectal Disease Symposium, Ft Lauderdale, Florida, February 13–15, 2003
2. Boccasanta P, Venturi M, Stuto A, et-al. Stapled transanal rectal resection for outlet obstruction: a prospective, multicenter trial. Dis Colon Rectum 2004; 47: 1285–1297
3. Mathur P, Ng K-H, Seow-Choen F.Stapled mucosectomy for rectocele repair: a preliminary report. Dis Colon Rectum 2004; 47: 1978–1981
4. Corman ML, Carriero A, Hager T, Herold A. Jayne DG, Lehur P-A, Lomanto, Longo A, Mellgren AF, Nicholls J, Nystrom P-O, Senagore AJ, Stuto A and Wexner SD. Consensus conference on the stapled transanal rectal resection (STARR) for disordered defecation. Colorectal Dis 2006; 8: 98–101
5. Jayne DG and Finan PJ. Stapled transanal rectal resection for obstructed defaecation and evidence-based practice. Br J Surg 2005; 92: 793–794
6. Renzi A, Izzo D, Di Sarno G, Izzo G, Di Martino N. Stapled transanal rectal resection to treat obstructed defecation caused by rectal intussusception and rectocele. Int J Colorectal Dis 2006; 21: 661–667
7. Petersen S, Hellmich G, Schuster A, Lehmann D, Albert W, Ludwig K. Stapled transanal rectal resection under laparoscopic surveillance for rectocele and concomitant enterocele. Dis Colon Rectum 2006; 49:1–5
8. Sielaff M, Scherer R, Gogler H, Farke S. Die STARR-Operation. Erfahrungen bei 60 patienten. Coloproctology 2006; 28: 217–223
9. Dodi G, Pietroletti R, Milito G, Binda G, Pescatori M. Bleeding, incontinence, pain and constipation after STARR transanal double stapling rectotomy for obstructed defecation. Tech Coloproctology 2003; 7: 148–153

Chapter 8
The Evidence for Stapled Hemorrhoidopexy and STARR

F.H. Hetzer and A. Senagore

Abstract Few areas of coloproctology attract as much attention or inspire so much heated debate than that of the treatment of hemorrhoids. Opinion varies widely and is frequently based on personal preference rather than a critical analysis of the literature. In this chapter an extensive review of the current literature on stapled hemorrhoidopexy and STARR is presented together with an overview of the current evidence level and grade of recommendation for both procedures. The reader is invited to assimilate the information provided and to come to an independent opinion on the relative merits of PPH and STARR, based on the best available scientific evidence.

Stapled Hemorrhoidopexy (PPH)

Introduction

Stapled hemorrhoidopexy has been hailed as a significant breakthrough in the surgical treatment of hemorrhoids. A first description of the use of a circular stapler device for the excision of hemorrhoids can be found in the work of Kobladin and Schalkow in Kazakhstan in 1981 [1]. In Europe, Allegra from Firenze published his experience with this new technique in 1990 [2]. However, Antonio Longo from Sicily modified and standardized the technique and became the advocate of the circular suturing device for the treatment of hemorrhoids in 1998 [3]. The procedure was steadily adopted by other surgeons and has been accepted worldwide as an effective treatment for advanced hemorrhoidal disease. Despite the reported successful outcomes with stapled hemorrhoidopexy, there have been reports of chronic pain and stricture formation in a small percentage of patients.

Probably no other surgical technique has been so thoroughly evaluated by the surgical community. There have been a large number of prospective randomized trials which have generally shown good results [4–37]. Similar information is available from case series [38–53], consensus papers [54–57], and systemic reviews [26, 58–63]. There have been several descriptions of technical modifications aimed at improving the outcomes or ease of performance [64–71]. Finally, there have also been case reports of complications [72–95] and recommendations on management options [47, 75, 82, 96–100]. In this chapter we will review the current body of evidence with regard to the procedure, including optimal techniques and evidence-based management to reduce complication rates. In accordance with the consensus paper from Corman et al. [55], we will refer to the technique as stapled hemorrhoidopexy or PPH (procedure for prolapse and hemorrhoids), whereas in older publications the terms stapled hemorrhoidectomy and mucosectomy have been used.

The randomized trials referred to in this chapter have been summarized in Table 8.1. When considering this literature one should keep in mind the level and grade of the evidence presented (Tables 8.2 and 8.3).

D. Jayne and A. Stuto (eds.), *Transanal Stapling Techniques for Anorectal Prolapse*,
DOI: 10.1007/978-1-84800-905-9_8, © Springer-Verlag London Limited 2009

TABLE 8.1. Randomized clinical trials comparing PPH with conventional hemorrhoidectomy.

Study	Year	Stage	PPH	Comparator	Median follow-up (months)	Conclusion
Mehigan et al. [17]	2000	PH	20	20 MM	4	Equal for: Symptomatic and Functional outcome PPH: with short-term benefit: Reduced pain Earlier recovery
Smyth et al. [25], follow-up on long-term results of Mehigan et al.	2003	PH	20	16 MM	37	Equal for: QoL Symptomatic and Functional outcome
Roswell et al. [22]	2000	III	11	11 Closed	1.5	PPH: with short-term benefit: Reduced pain Shorter length of stay Earlier recovery
Au-Yong et al. [4], follow-up on long-term results by Roswell et al.	2004	III	11	9 Closed	42	Equal for: Recurrence rate Functional outcome
Ho et al. [14]	2000	III/IV	57	62 MM	5	Equal for: Length of stay Functional outcome Patient satisfaction and QoL PPH: with short-term benefit: Reduced pain Symptomatic outcome Earlier recovery MM: causes less costs
Ooi et al. [28], follow-up on long-term results by Ho et al.	2002	III and IV	33	27	17	Equal for: Recurrence rate Functional outcome
Helmy [11]	2000	PH	20	20 MM	3	Equal for: Functional and symptomatic outcome Length of stay PPH: with short-term benefit: Reduced pain Earlier recovery
Boccasanta et al. [5]	2001	IV	40	40 HLB	20	Equal for: Functional and symptomatic outcome PPH: with short-term benefit: Reduced pain Length of stay Earlier recovery
Ganio et al. [10]	2001	III and IV	50	50 MM	16	PPH: with short-term benefit: Reduced pain Better functional outcome Shorter length of stay Earlier recovery
Ganio et al. [101], follow-up on long-term results by Ganio et al.	2007	III and IV	40	37 MM	87	Equal for: Functional and symptomatic outcome
Shalaby et al. [24]	2001	II–IV	100	100 MM	12	PPH: with short-term benefit: Reduced pain Symptomatic and functional outcome Shorter length of stay Earlier recovery

HLB Hospital Leopold Bellan (modified Milligan–Morgan) Multicenter trial

Closed = Mucosal wound closed, but skin wound left open

Study	Year	Grade	N	N	Months	Outcome	Comments
Brown et al. [6]	2001	tPH	15	16 MM	1.5	PPH: with benefit: Reduced pain Symptomatic outcome Earlier recovery	tPH = acute thrombosed circumferentially prolapsed piles
Pavlidis et al. [20]	2002	II–IV	40	40 MM	3	Equal for: Functional and symptomatic outcome PPH: with short-term benefit: Reduced pain Length of stay Patient satisfaction	
Hetzer et al. [12]	2002	II and III	20	20 FH	12	Equal for: Functional and symptomatic outcome Length of stay PPH: with short-term benefit: Reduced pain Earlier recovery	
Correa-Rovelo et al. [9]	2002	III and IV	42	42 FH	7–14	Equal for: Patient satisfaction FH: better symptomatic outcome PPH: with short-term benefit: Reduced pain Earlier recovery	
Wilson et al. [27]	2002	III	59*	30 MM	1.5–2	Equal for: Length of stay QoL PPH: with short-term benefit: Earlier recovery MM: with less postoperative bleeding	*27 Autosuture and 32 Ethicon stapled; hemorrhoidopexy; Multicenter trial
Ortiz et al. [102]	2002	III and IV	27	28 MM	16	Equal for: Length of stay Recovery PPH: with short-term benefit: Earlier recovery MM: with less recurrence	
Kairaluoma et al. [15]	2003	III	30	30 MM	12	Equal for: Length of stay Recovery Patient satisfaction PPH: with short-term benefit: Reduced pain MM: with better functional outcome	Day-case setting
Peng et al. [103]	2003	III and IV	30	25 RB	6	Equal for: QoL Functional outcome Patient satisfaction PPH: with more pain and complications RB with more recurrent bleeding	RB rubber band ligation
Palimento et al. [19]	2003	III and IV	37	37 MM	6	Equal for: Functional outcome Recovery Patient satisfaction PPH: with short-term benefit: Reduced pain	Multicenter Trial
Picchio et al. [29], follow-up on long-term results by Palimento et al.	2003	III and IV	37	37 MM	42	Equal for: Functional and symptomatic outcome Patient satisfaction	Telephone interview
Cheetham et al. [7]	2003	PH	15	16 MM	6	Equal for: Recovery PPH: with short-term benefit: Reduced pain MM: with better mid-term outcome Functional and symptomatic outcome	
Krska et al. [30]	2003	III	25	25 MM	1	PPH: with short-term benefit: Reduced pain Shorter length of stay Lower CRP and fibrinogen levels	

(continued)

TABLE 8.1. (continued)

Study	Year	Stage	PPH	Comparator	Median follow-up (months)	Conclusion	
Racalbuto et al. [21]	2004	III and IV	50	50 MM	48	PPH: with short-term benefit: Reduced pain Shorter length of stay	
Senagore et al. [23]	2004	III	77	79 FH	12	Equal for: Functional and symptomatic outcome	Multicenter Trial
Lau et al. [31]	2004	II and III	13	11 MM	2	PPH: with short-term benefit: Reduced pain Shorter length of stay Less follow-up interventions Equal for: Pain PPH: Shorter length of stay MM: Better reduction of skin tags	
Bikhchandani et al. [32]	2004	III and IV	42	42 MM	11	Equal for: Complications PPH: with short-term benefit: Reduced pain Shorter length of stay Patient satisfaction Earlier recovery	
Basdanis et al. [33]	2005	III and IV	50	45 MM	18	Equal for: Functional outcome Costs PPH: with short-term benefit: Reduced pain Earlier recovery	MM with Ligasure
Ortiz et al. [18]	2005	IV	15	16 MM	12	PPH was not effective in fourth-degree hemorrhoids and was responsible for tenesmus in 40% of the patients	
Chung et al. [8]	2005	III	43	45 MM	6	PPH with short-term benefit: Reduced pain Shorter length of stay Earlier recovery	MM with Harmonic Scalpel
Gravie et al. [34]	2005	SH	63	63 MM	24	Equal for: Functional and symptomatic outcome PPH: with short-term benefit: Reduced pain during defecation Shorter length of stay Earlier recovery	Multicenter Trial
Kraemer et al. [16]	2005	II–IV	25	25 MM	1.5	Equal for: Pain Patient satisfaction Recovery MM: better control in fourth-degree	Multicenter trial; MM with Ligasure
Van de Stadt et al. [104]	2005	II and III	20	20 MM	46	PPH with a higher recurrence rate Equal for: Patient satisfaction	
Ho et al. [13]	2006	III and IV	29	21 FH	8.5	PPH with short-term benefit: Reduced pain Shorter length of stay Better symptomatic outcome	
Mattana et al. [105]	2007	IV	50	50 MM	54/92	MM with benefit: Resumption of symptoms Risk of recurrence	

PH prolapsing hemorrhoids; SH symptomatic hemorrhoids; PPH procedure for prolapse and hemorrhoids; MM Milligan–Morgan; FH Ferguson hemorrhoidectomy. Functional outcome includes: incontinence, constipation, and stenosis. Symptomatic outcome includes symptoms, such as bleeding, itching, prolapsing mucosa, related to internal hemorrhoids

TABLE 8.2. Definitions of evidence levels and grades of recommendation, according to Cook and Sackett [106, 107].

Level I	Evidence obtained from meta-analysis of multiple well-designed controlled studies; randomized trials with low false-positive and false-negative errors (high power)
Level II	Evidence obtained from at least one well-designed experimental study; randomized trials with high false-positive and false-negative errors or both (low power)
Level III	Evidence obtained from well-designed, quasiexperimental studies, such as nonrandomized, controlled, single-group, preoperative/postoperative comparison, cohort, time, or matched case-control series
Level IV	Evidence obtained from well-designed no experimental studies, such as comparative and correlational descriptive and case studies
Level V	Evidence obtained from case reports and clinical examples
Grade A	Evidence of level I or consistent findings from multiple studies of levels II, III, or IV
Grade B	Evidence of levels II, III, or IV; findings are generally consistent
Grade C	Evidence of levels II, III, or IV; findings are inconsistent
Grade D	Little or no systematic empiric evidence

TABLE 8.3. Evidence level and grade of recommendation as applied to the literature on the PPH-procedure.

	Evidence level and grade of recommendation
Grade II and III hemorrhoids	I/A
Grade IV hemorrhoids	I/C
Rectal varices	V/D
Day-case setting	IV/C
Perioperative antibiotics	V/D
Postoperative flavonoids	V/D
Albumin-glutaraldehyde bioadhesive "Bioglue"	II/D
Control of bleeding: PPH03 > PPH01	II/B
Double purse string	II/D
Two staple lines	V/D

Patient Selection

Most authors agree that PPH is most effective for treating symptoms in third degree or prolapsing hemorrhoids. Treating fourth-degree hemorrhoids by PPH has generally been less effective and associated with higher recurrence rates [16, 18, 108]. Obviously, earlier stage disease can be more cost effectively managed by injection or rubber band ligation, and PPH is not indicated in such cases [103]. PPH has also been described for the safe and successful treatment of rectal varices [109–111].

There has been concern that the large-diameter circular anal dilator required for insertion of the purse-string suture and insertion of the intraluminal stapler may produce internal anal sphincter injuries [80, 93]. This risk has not been supported by preoperative/postoperative comparative studies which have focused on anorectal physiology assessment or incontinence scoring [10, 12, 14, 102, 103, 112]. However, because symptomatic sphincter dysfunction may occur many years after the injury, it is recommended that surgeons perform gentle anal dilation with adjunctive anal sphincter blockade with local anesthetic [113]. Patients with pre-existing sphincter damage should be counseled about the risk of worsening continence postoperatively.

Appropriate counseling should be given before recommending PPH to patients who practice anal intercourse [114, 115]. After PPH, a circular line of staples is left in the anal canal with the potential risk of penile injury or condom damage. Although the staples are rarely visible 3 months after the operation, the staple line is still palpable and can cause discomfort or injury during intercourse and may be a source of medical litigation [115].

The PPH Technique and Its Modifications

The applicability of PPH to day-case surgery has been described, and its use in this setting appears to be dominated more by the economics of the health care system rather than surgical outcomes [7, 15, 49, 116–119]. Most of the procedures were performed under general [5–7, 9, 10, 12, 14, 15, 17, 22, 24, 37, 44, 49, 93, 120–122], spinal, or epidural anesthesia [5, 10, 12, 18–20, 30, 37, 93, 120–122]. Peridural saddle anesthesia [21] and anal block [21, 23, 118, 123–125] are also options. Concomitant intraoperative infiltration of adrenaline and local anesthetic were used in a few trials [10, 11, 15, 17, 21, 22, 24]. PPH is generally performed faster than excisional hemorrhoidectomy, which together with the reduced postoperative pain, makes it an effective day-case procedure [7, 10].

Prophylactic antibiotics were used in about half of the published studies [5, 7, 9, 11, 12, 17, 18, 20, 22, 24, 102]. This may require further investigation following the report by Maw et al. who describes an 11% rate of bacteremia following PPH compared to 5% after diathermy hemorrhoidectomy [126]. The isolated organisms were predominantly anaerobes commonly found within the bacterial flora of the anorectum [5–7, 9, 10, 12, 17, 19, 20, 22, 24, 27, 30, 102, 127].

The use of flavonoids (micronized purified flavonoid fraction) to reduce bleeding and pain after conventional hemorrhoidectomy has been recommended in three studies [128–130]. However, the benefit could not be reproduced in the only randomized controlled study with PPH [99].

Perez-Vicente et al. recommended a double purse string for PPH in order to resect a greater doughnut of distal rectal mucosa. Their prospective randomized controlled trial demonstrated that they increased the distance of the staple line from the dentate line and reduced early postoperative pain in comparison to a single purse-string technique [131]. Long-term benefits associated with this modification have not been reported.

The new PPH03 stapler seems to be more effective than the PPH01 stapler in controlling bleeding from the staple line suture, as reported in one randomized controlled study [132] and in several case series [133, 134].

The use of a linear cutter instead of a circular stapler was described by Khalil et al. [135]. The procedure demonstrated less postoperative pain compared to closed hemorrhoidectomy; however, no comparison was made with the PPH technique.

Albumin-glutaraldehyde bioadhesive ("Bioglue") was used in a single randomized controlled trial and recommended by Anghelacopoulos et al. for the prevention of postoperative complications after PPH. The authors found that patients who received Bioglue had no complications compared to the control group (no Bioglue) in which there were two cases of anal stenosis, two postoperative bleeds, three postoperative leaks, and one thrombosis [64].

The feasibility and safety of repeat PPH for recurrent prolapse has not been described in the literature. However, Zmora et al. investigated the feasibility and safety of a second stapler resection

close to the initial line in an animal model [136]. The mucosal blood flow between the two staple lines and the degree of fibrosis did not differ significantly from the flow measured in the proximal rectum, suggesting the possibility of ischemic complications was low.

Various modifications to the instrumentation have been described, primarily to improve surgical access to the anal canal. Modifications to the anoscope for improved purse-string insertion, and the anal dilators to accommodate various body types have all been proposed [65, 68, 137–139]. The use of a Deaver retractor has been suggested to allow better visualization of the staple line [140]. There has also been a device for purse-string placement without using an anoscope [69].

Eversion of the anal canal with or without the use of the LoneStar™ retractor has been suggested by several authors as a means of avoiding excessive anal sphincter stretching by the circular anal dilator [66, 71].

Clinical Outcomes Following PPH

The majority of the short-term trials have found that stapled hemorrhoidopexy is less painful and that the complication rate is either lower or the same as conventional hemorrhoidectomy.

Pain

Randomized trials of the PPH procedure almost invariably show that it is associated with significantly less postoperative pain compared to conventional surgery [5, 7–12, 14–20, 22–24, 30–34, 102]. This appears to be true for pain at rest as well as pain associated with defecation [34]. PPH does however cause more pain compared to rubber band ligation [103].

Histological Assessment

Attempts to explain the risk of postoperative pain on staple line location have focused on the presence of squamous epithelium within the resection specimen. Ohana et al. suggested that the presence of only squamous epithelium in the resected tissue was significantly associated with severe postoperative pain persisting greater than 1 week after surgery [44]. However, the presence of both squamous and glandular epithelium correlated only with severe pain on the first postoperative day. Several studies have reported the presence of internal sphincter muscle [22, 31, 135, 141, 142] and even external anal sphincter muscle in the post-PPH specimen [135]. Despite these findings, there appears to be little correlation with postoperative incontinence. Lau et al. did report that the presence of smooth muscle correlated with a reduction in the maximum squeeze pressure on manometry. However, they felt this reduction was more closely related to excessive dilatation by the 37-mm circular anal dilator (CAD) [31]. A randomized trial, however, did associate a higher incidence of sphincter fragmentation with the use of the anal dilator than without [14].

Anorectal Physiology

Published anorectal physiology data on the effect of PPH on sphincter function have shown mixed results. No significant change was noted in the majority of the trials [10, 14, 18, 103, 112, 141]. However, one study noted a significant decrease in postoperative pressure following diathermy excision [24], and a separate study showed reduced maximal squeeze pressure after PPH [31]. A separate study identified a significant reduction in anal resting pressure in the PPH-treated group when a Parks retractor was used [143].

Recovery

The systemic review of Tjandra et al. published in 2007 [61] confirmed a significantly shorter time to first bowel movement [9, 16, 18, 23, 32, 34, 102], duration of hospital stay [5, 8, 10–12, 14–17, 20–24, 27, 30–34], time off work [5, 8, 9, 12, 30, 32, 102], and return to normal activities [14, 21, 22, 24, 33, 34, 144] with PPH. As mentioned previously, both PPH and excisional hemorrhoidectomy can be safely used in the day-case setting. PPH allowed a faster functional recovery with 7 days earlier return to work and 16 days earlier return to normal activities [61]. These results may be related to faster wound healing following PPH as compared to conventional hemorrhoidectomy (0% unhealed vs. 11.2%) [7, 9, 12, 14, 22, 33]. The staple line height (>22 mm) was inversely related to return to work and narcotic usage in the study by Plocek et al. [98].

Patient Satisfaction

Significantly more patients have rated PPH with greater satisfaction as compared to conventional hemorrhoidectomy in randomized controlled studies [11, 17, 19, 20, 22, 24, 32, 144].

Quality of Life

Three randomized, controlled trials have addressed the quality of life using the SF-36 [25, 27] and Eypasch questionnaires [14], and found no significant between PPH and excisional hemorrhoidectomy. One nonrandomized trial has reported a significant benefit following PPH at 6-month follow-up [121].

Complications

The overall complication rates are comparable in both procedures: 20.2% for PPH and 25.2% for conventional hemorrhoidectomy [61]. However, PPH has been associated with less postoperative bleeding [7, 9–11, 14–17, 20, 21, 24, 27, 30, 33, 102, 145], wound problems [7, 9–13, 17, 23, 24, 30, 32, 33, 102], constipation [9, 10, 14, 18, 20, 21, 23, 27, 30, 34, 102], and pruritus [9, 14, 23]. The rates of postoperative external hemorrhoidal thrombosis [5, 8, 9, 12, 14, 18, 24, 30, 34, 102], residual anal skin tags [5, 11, 14, 21, 24, 34], fecal incontinence [5, 8–12, 14, 17, 21, 23, 30, 31, 33, 34], urgency of stool [7–9, 15, 17, 21, 23], early [9, 15, 23, 30, 34, 88] or late [5, 9, 12, 14–17, 19, 21, 22, 24, 30, 92] stenosis, anal fissure [7, 16, 17, 19, 21, 23, 24, 34], perianal fistula [12, 19, 21, 23, 102], rectovaginal fistulas [146, 147] and urinary retention were similar. Importantly, the reintervention rate (nonsurgical [5, 7–12, 14, 15, 17, 18, 21, 23, 24, 27, 31, 32, 34, 102] and surgical [5, 7–10, 12, 14, 15, 17–24, 27, 30, 32, 34, 102]) and the readmission rate [7, 14, 17, 34] is similar for PPH and excisional hemorrhoidectomy. In not randomized studies the reintervention rate varies from 0 to 6% [93, 120, 148, 149].

There has been a single report of complete staple closure of the rectum with PPH. It is likely that this complication is under-reported [150], but it should be avoidable with careful attention to the correct placement of the purse-string suture. If it does occur, it should be immediately obvious on inspection of the staple line and correctable at the time of surgery.

A low hemorrhoidopexy staple line is associated with increased postoperative pain [151–153], prolonged recovery time [98], and may increase the risk of incontinence [97, 142]. Conversely, a staple line >40 mm above the dentate line increases the risk of persistent or recurrent hemorrhoidal prolapse. Therefore, Williams et al. recommend a staple line between 20 and 40 mm above dental line [154].

Pescatori reported six patients with chronic pain after PPH, related to a painful rectal intramucosal pocket with an endoluminal orifice at the suture line: the "rectal pocket syndrome." Four of these patients needed revisional surgery [87].

Severe intraperitoneal bleeding due to a deep enterocele has been reported in a patient after PPH by Aumann et al. [72], and in a two other cases following resection of rectal lesions [73, 155]. Perirectal hematoma and hypovolemic shock after rectal stapled mucosectomy for hemorrhoids have been described by others [156].

Fournier's gangrene is a well-known and often fatal fasciitis of the pelvic floor following anorectal, urologic, and gynecologic procedures. Although rare, both Fournier's gangrene and pelvic sepsis have been reported in association with PPH [84, 85, 89, 91, 157–161], with at least one mortality PPH [74]. Interestingly, one anecdotal case described a chicken bone perforation as the cause of late-onset anal abscess after PPH [81].

Pneumoretroperitoneum, pneumomediastinum, and subcutaneous emphysema of the neck after stapled hemorrhoidopexy have been reported by Filingeri et al. [77] and following dilatation of a PPH-induced stricture by Kanellos [83].

Recurrence Rate

One area of continuing controversy when comparing PPH and conventional hemorrhoidectomy is the rate of recurrent prolapse. Some studies have reported no difference in the rates of early recurrence (recurrence within 6 months) between the two techniques [7–9, 15, 16, 22, 23]. In contrast, other studies have suggested an increased rate of recurrent prolapse following PPH [7, 9, 10, 14, 17–24, 34, 102]. The 2007 systematic review by Tjandra et al. showed a 5.7 recurrence rate at 1 year following PPH compared to 1% following hemorrhoidectomy [61]. This was matched by a nonsignificant trend

toward more recurrent hemorrhoidal symptoms following PPH ($p = 0.07$).

The findings of Tjandra et al. have subsequently been confirmed by the meta-analysis performed on behalf of NICE in 2007 [162]. This reported a nonsignificant trend to early recurrent prolapse after PPH (relative risk < 1 year = 3.20), but a significant increased incidence on long-term follow-up (relative risk > 1 year = 4.34). Thus, there would appear to be two components to recurrent prolapse: early recurrence associated with inadequate excision at the time of original surgery, and "true" late recurrence despite a previously adequate resection. These findings have led some authors to conclude that PPH has limited efficacy for large volume, fourth-degree hemorrhoids, and therefore conventional hemorrhoidectomy has been recommended [16, 18, 108].

Cost Effectiveness

Only a few trials [5, 14, 27, 33, 163] have investigated cost effectiveness, and all but one found no significant difference comparing PPH with conventional hemorrhoidectomy. In the Asian study the cost was higher for the PPH despite earlier recovery and return to work [11]. The 2007 NICE appraisal compared the short-term costs of stapled hemorrhoidopexy with conventional hemorrhoidectomy at 3-month follow-up [162]. Although the operative cost of the stapled procedure was more expensive, due mainly to the price of the stapler, this was largely offset by a shorter length of hospital stay. Overall, stapled hemorrhoidopexy was marginally more expensive, but at only an additional £19 per case. It was noted that the economic model used was sensitive to minor changes, particularly in the cost of utilities. In addition, the analysis did not take into account any cost savings arising from the decreased wound complication rate and earlier recovery following PPH. The report concluded that "stapled hemorrhoidopexy might lead to modest cost saving" and that "stapled hemorrhoidopexy would be an appropriate use of NHS resources."

Conclusion

Stapled hemorrhoidopexy offers significant advantages, at least in respect to short-term outcomes and patient satisfaction, provided patients with symptomatic prolapsing piles are appropriately selected. Complications are generally lower for PPH compared to conventional hemorrhoidectomy. Data from a large number of randomized studies and meta-analyses suggest that PPH is safe and a cost-effective treatment. It appears that PPH may be associated with a higher long-term risk of hemorrhoid recurrence, especially prolapse. It is also likely to be associated with a higher risk of long-term symptom recurrence, and the need for reintervention compared to conventional hemorrhoidectomy. A summary of the evidence to date, comparing the outcomes after stapled hemorrhoidopexy with conventional hemorrhoidectomy, is presented in Table 8.4.

Further long-term follow-up data are required to determine whether these findings are a technical or disease-specific issue.

Stapled Transanal Rectal Resection

Stapled transanal rectal resection (STARR) was first described by Dr. Antonio Longo as a novel surgical treatment for obstructed defecation syndrome (ODS) [164]. The clinical and experimental observations that led to the development of STARR have been described in Chap. 1. The technique uses a circular stapler to produce a full-thickness circumferential of the distal rectum. The aim is to excise any redundancy of the distal rectum, manifest

Table 8.4. Evidence for PPH procedure compared to conventional hemorrhoidectomy. *PPH* procedure for prolapse and hemorrhoids; *CH* conventional hemorrhoidectomy

	Favoring PPH			Favoring CH	
Variable	Significant	Tendency	Equal	Tendency	Significant
Operating time	I/A				
Postoperative pain	I/A				
Recovery					
First bowel movement	I/A				
Hospital stay	I/A				
Return to work	I/A				
Return to normal activities	I/A				
Patient's satisfaction	I/A				
Quality of life		II/B			
Complications			I/A		
Bleeding	I/A				
Urinary retention	I/A				
Wound problems	I/A				
Pruritus	I/A				
Perianal thrombosis			I/A		
Residual anal skin tag			I/A		
Recurrent prolapse			I/A		
Stenosis		I/A			
Fissure		I/A			
Fistula		I/A			
Reinterventions		I/A			
Readmissions		I/A			
Bowel function					
Constipation	I/A				
Incontinence		I/A			
Urge at stool		I/A			
Recurrence					
Early recurrence (<6 months)				I/A	
Late recurrence					I/A
Cost effectiveness		II/C			

as rectocele or internal prolapse/intussusception, which is believed to be the causative factor responsible for ODS.

The evidence for STARR in the published literature remains limited, being restricted to small randomized trials and personal case series (Table 8.5). This fact hindered the 2006 National Institute for Health and Clinical Excellence (NICE) assessment of STARR and resulted in the issuing of cautious guidance. This stated "current evidence on the safety and efficacy of stapled transanal rectal resection (STARR) does not appear adequate for this procedure to be used without special arrangements and for audit or research" [179]. On the back of this guidance, a collaborative initiative between Italy, Germany, and Great Britain, the European STARR Registry, was established with specific aims to audit the short-term safety and efficacy of STARR.

TABLE 8.5. Published clinical trials for stapled transanal rectal resection (STARR) for obstructed defecation syndrome (ODS) or rectal prolapse. *CCS-Score* Cleveland Clinic Constipation Score [165]

Study	Year	STARR	Comparator	Median follow-up (months)	CCS-Score pre/post		Conclusion	Comments
Dodi et al. [166]	2003	14	No	12	No	No	Success rate: 50% in ODS	
							Severe complications, pain, bleeding, fecal incontinence	
							Early recurrence	
Boccasanta et al. [167]	2004	90	No	16	13.0	4.5	Good results in 90% in ODS	Multicenter trial
							Safe and effective technique	
Boccasanta et al. [168]	2004	25	25 STAPL	23	18.0	5.7	In ODS 88% good results for STARR, 76% for STAPL	Randomized controlled trial; *STAPL* stapled trans-anal prolapsectomy with perineal levatorplasty
							Equal for: Safety and effectiveness	
							STARR with Less pain Absence of dysperunia Better reduction of the rectocele	
Schwandner et al. [169]	2005	16	No	6	18.6	3.8	Success rate: 93% in ODS	
							Safe and effective technique	
Ommer et al. [170]	2006	14	No	19	13	4	Success rate: 93% in ODS	Defecation score [171]
							Safe and effective	
Renzi et al. [172]	2006	71	No	6	17.0	7.9	Success rate: 90% in ODS	
							Safe and effective technique	
Sielaff et al. [173]	2006	60	No	16	12.7	6.6	Success rate 67% in ODS	
							Cave pre-existing fecal incontinence	
Arroyo et al. [174]	2007	37	No	24	12.7	4.1	Success rate: 95% in ODS	
							Safe and effective technique	

(continued)

TABLE 8.5. (continued)

Study	Year	STARR	Comparator	Median follow-up (months)	CCS-Score pre/post		Conclusion	Comments
Boccasanta et al. [145]	2007	34	34 SA	8	5.1	2.9	Equal for: Hospital stay Morbidity Time to return to normal activity STARR with More transient fecal urgency Better reduction of rectal prolapse	Randomized controlled trial; *SA* stapled anopexy
Pechlivanides et al. [175]	2007	37	No	9	9.5	3.0	Success rate: 88% in ODS Safe and effective technique	17 STARR procedures with PPH01 and 20 with PPH03
Boccasanta et al. [176]	2008	10	No	27	14.7	3.0	Success rate: 80% Minimal complications, no recurrence	Rectal ulcer associated with rectal prolapsed
Gagliardi et al. [177]	2008	85	No	17			Improvement: 65% High morbidity (bleeding): 12% High reoperation rate: 19% Recurrence rate: 11%	
Frascio et al. [178]	2008	25	No	25	–	–	Success rate: 76%	

Publication of the 1-year follow-up results from the Registry is expected by the end of 2008.

Previous attempts to resect rectoceles and concomitant rectal prolapse using a single 33-mm circular stapler (PPH01) have been described by Pescatori et al. in 1997 [180]. A combined procedure incorporating perineal repair with a stapled transanal resection was described by Altomare et al. in 2002 [181]. Antonio Longo further developed his idea to include the use of two staplers to produce a circumferential rectal resection by means of separate anterior and posterior firings of the stapler [166] A multicenter trial in 2004 demonstrated the safety and efficacy of this approach [167]. Other single-center studies followed [166–170, 172–175], and in 2005 the first consensus paper on STARR for ODS was published [182]. Only two randomized controlled trials [145, 168] have been performed. In two of these, Boccasanta et al. compared Longo's STARR procedure with the technique described by Altomare in 2002 [181] and Pescatori in 1997 [180], and found that both were effective in reducing ODS symptoms but that STARR was preferable in terms of reduced postoperative pain, absence of dysperunia, and correction of rectocele on postoperative proctography [145].

Patient Selection

In all but one of the published studies [145] ODS is cited as the indication for the STARR procedure. The one study where STARR was used for an alternative indication was that by Boccassanta et al., where STARR was used in patients with symptomatic hemorrhoids associated with rectal prolapse; in this study, STARR was found to be more effective than conventional stapled hemorrhoidopexy.

Concern has been raised about the use of STARR in patients with sphincter defects or impaired continence. In such circumstances, the rectal intussusception and associated outlet obstruction may mask impaired sphincter function, and its excision can potentially result in a worsening of continence [173]. This concern has never been formally investigated, but it has not materialized as an over-riding problem in clinical practice. This may be due to the fact that chronic straining and rectoanal intussusception in itself produces a degree of sphincter dilatation, which improves with subsequent excision of the offending prolapse. In addition, it has been learned from stapled hemorrhoidopexy that the large-diameter circular anal dilator, if applied carefully, can be used in patients with occult sphincter weakness without adverse effects on continence.

The STARR Technique and Its Modifications

In two studies STARR was performed as a day-case procedure [172, 174]. In other clinical trials, however, the hospital stay has varied from 2 to 7 days [167–170, 173]. Most of the procedures were performed under general [145, 166–170, 173, 174], spinal, or epidural anesthesia [145, 166–170, 172–174]. The operation duration in all studies ranges between 35 and 43 min [145, 167–169, 172–174]. Complete mechanical bowel preparation was recommended in three of eight studies [166, 173, 174], whereas the remaining reports recommend a simple enema immediately prior to surgery [145, 167–170]. Prophylactic antibiotics were used in the majority of the studies [166–170, 183].

All but one surgeon used two PPH01 staplers for STARR. Arroya et al. performed 17 STARR procedures with PPH01 and 20 with the PPH03. In this study the new PPH03 stapler device seems to be more effective than the PPH01 for control of bleeding; however, its use cannot be recommended due to the shorter staple height which may predispose to staple line dehiscence. It should be noted that the use of the PPH03 stapler for STARR is an "off-license" application.

Since October 2006 a new stapler has been available for STARR; the Contour Transtar, supplied as the STR5G kit. The set includes a 30-mm Contour Transtar stapler, an access suture anoscope, a 30-mm circular anal dilator and an obturator. The Contour Transtar was designed specifically for STARR and aimed to address some of the shortcomings of the double-stapled PPH-STARR technique. With the PPH-STARR

method, the PPH01 stapler was limited in the amount of rectal prolapse that could be resected due to capacity of the stapler housing. Use of the PPH01 also requires exclusion of the opposite rectal wall with a retractor, and the procedure was performed "blind" with no control over the extent of prolapse resection. In contrast, STARR performed with the Contour Transtar may improve visualization and provide the operator with a degree of discretion as to the amount of rectal tissue to resect. Although these advantages of the Contour Transtar appear to be apparent in clinical practice, there are no data comparing PPH01 STARR with Contour Transtar STARR. Likewise, there is no evidence as yet to support or refute the hypothesis that a bigger prolapse resection achievable with the Contour Transtar results in an improved functional outcome.

In patients with ODS and coexistent enterocele a laparoscopic-guided STARR has been recommended [183]. Laparoscopy allows direct visualization of the transanal resection with exclusion of the small bowel from the Pouch of Douglas. Incorporation of the peritoneal lining of the Pouch of Douglas within the Transtar resection may be effective in simultaneously dealing with the enterocele.

Results

Although the data on STARR remain relatively limited, the majority of the reports would suggest that there is a significant improvement in ODS symptoms with an acceptable complication profile.

Pain

The STARR procedure is associated with moderate postoperative pain, similar to that of stapled hemorrhoidopexy. The level of pain peaks by about the second postoperative day and with the patient being pain-free by around the tenth postoperative day [167, 168]. Occasional instances of protracted pain and persistent defecatory disorders have been reported [169].

Histological Assessment

In contrast to stapled hemorrhoidopexy, the STARR procedure produces a full-thickness resection of the distal rectum. Therefore rectal smooth-muscle fibers should be found in 100% of patients [167–169, 174]. Schwandner's group analyzed the resected tissue and found in three patients (18.8%) intestinal neuronal type B dysplasia by immuno-histochemistry [169].

Anorectal Physiology

Data concerning the effect of STARR on anorectal physiology have shown mixed results. No significant change in resting or squeeze pressures was noted by Boccasanta, Arroyo, and Renzi [167, 168, 172, 174]. However, Pechlivanides found a significant increase in the maximum resting anal pressure and a decrease in rectal compliance post-operatively [175].

Defecographic Assessment

Almost all studies have assessed patients preoperatively using dynamic defecography. Additionally, four studies performed comparative postoperative defecography. Pechilivanides et al. found a significant reduction in the anterior rectocele, intussusceptions, and perineal descent on straining [175]. Similar results have been reported by Renzi et al. [172]. Boccasanta and coworkers additionally described no evidence of entrapped contrast after defecation in 80–85% of patients following STARR [167, 168].

Recovery

The mean time for return to normal activity was only assessed in the randomized controlled trial by Bocassanta in 2007 [145]. In this study, the STARR procedure was performed for hemorrhoidal disease with concomitant rectal prolapse. The mean time to return to normal activity was 14 days.

Patient Satisfaction

A wide range of patient satisfaction is reported following STARR. However, most studies have demonstrated excellent or good levels of satisfaction (37% Sielaff; 57% Ommers [170], 80% Schwandener [169] and Renzi [172], 88% Boccasanta [167] and Pechlivanides [175]). Completely unsatisfied patients with poor outcomes have been found in 0–20% of patients depending upon the definitions used.

Quality of Life

Limited data exist regarding quality of life (QoL) following STARR. Few studies have included a formal QoL assessment using validated and recognized tools. However, most studies have used the Cleveland Clinic Constipation Score to quantify outcome, which does include a limited assessment of the impact of constipation symptoms on daily function (Table 8.5), and have shown a significant decrease in overall constipation scores. This is an area that requires further research, particularly when one considers that ODS is a benign condition and that the primary impact is on QoL.

Complications

A wide range of complication rates have been reported following STARR, ranging from 0% [169] at one extreme, to around 16% in the majority of studies [167, 168, 170, 172–174, 177], to 38% [166] at the other extreme. The most frequently reported early complications include acute urinary retention [145, 166, 168, 172], urinary infection [173], and rectal bleeding [145, 168, 170, 172–174, 177]. One patient was treated with antibiotics for perianal sepsis [166]. Late complications include rectal stenosis [166–168, 172, 173], protracted defecatory urgency [167, 168], rectal diverticulum [184] or pain [166, 170, 173, 177], and fecal incontinence [166–168, 173, 177]. Sielaff performed four reinterventions to remove retained staples, although the rationale for this was not clearly explained. A rectovaginal fistula after a STARR procedure was reported in 2006 by Bassi et al. [185]. The fistula occurred 3 weeks after the operation, which was complicated by a hematoma of the posterior vaginal wall. Gagliardi et al. reported three interventions with colostomy due to fistulas [177]. Interestingly, Li Destri et al. [186] recently described a rectovaginal fistula repair by a closure of the rectal opening with the STARR technique. Although the incidence of dysperunia has been evaluated in most studies, it has never been reported as a complication [145, 167–169, 172].

Recurrence Rate

Currently, the length of follow-up in most studies is not sufficient to determine with any degree of accuracy the true rate of ODS recurrence following STARR. Most

TABLE 8.6. Evidence level for different perioperative aspects of the STARR procedure [106, 107].

	Evidence level and grade of recommendation
Obstructed defecation syndrome	IV/B
Rectal prolapse	V/D
Day-case setting	IV/D
Perioperative antibiotics	IV/B
Bowel preparation	IV/D
Control of bleeding: PPH03 > PPH01	V/D
Laparoscopic-assistance	V/D

studies include a short-term (<12 months) or mid-term (<5 years) follow-up. Arroyo from Spain reported 2(5.4%) recurrences at 2-year follow-up [174] and Gagliardi 9(11%) [177] at 17 months. Ommer from Germany had a single male patient with increased symptoms 4 months postoperatively [170].

Cost Effectiveness

No study has included an analysis of cost effectiveness in relation to STARR. Given the fact that previous treatments for STARR, such as the internal Delorme's procedure, involved minimal operative costs this area needs to be formally evaluated. It may be that the cost of the staplers used in STARR, similar to the case for stapled hemorrhoidopexy, will be offset by a reduction in the length of hospital stay. However, this hypothesis will be difficult to assess given that few surgeons would now be happy performing an internal Delorme's for ODS.

Conclusion

The evidence concerning the safety and efficacy of STARR is based on a few case series, one multi-center study, and two small randomized controlled trials. Therefore, evidence levels and grades of recommendation are limited (Table 8.6). Randomized controlled trials, with long-term follow-up data, are required to formally evaluate STARR and to determine its position within the treatment algorithm of obstructed defecation. These studies should include an assessment of quality of life and cost effectiveness.

References

1. Koblandin SN and Schalkow JL. (1981) "Eine neue Methode zur Behandlung von Hämorrhoiden mit Hilfe eines Zirkularstaplers". Kasachstan: Wissenschaftliches Archiv des Zelinograder Medizinischen Institutes, pp 27–28.
2. Allegra G. (1990) [Experiences with mechanical staplers: hemorrhoidectomy using a circular stapler]. G. Chir. 11:95–97.
3. Longo A. (1998) Treatment of haemorrhoid disease by reduction of mucosa an haemorrhoidal prolapse with a circular suturing device: a new procedure. In: Proceedings of the 6th World Congress of Endoscopic Surgery. Bologna, Italy: Monduzzi Publishing Co, pp 777–784.
4. Au-Yong I, Rowsell M, Hemingway DM. (2004) Randomised controlled clinical trial of stapled haemorrhoidectomy vs conventional haemorrhoidectomy; a three and a half year follow up. Colorectal Dis. 6:37–38.
5. Boccasanta P, Capretti PG, Venturi M, Cioffi U, et al. (2001) Randomised controlled trial between stapled circumferential mucosectomy and conventional circular hemorrhoidectomy in advanced hemorrhoids with external mucosal prolapse. Am. J. Surg. 182:64–68.
6. Brown SR, Ballan K, Ho E, Ho Fams YH, et al. (2001) Stapled mucosectomy for acute thrombosed circumferentially prolapsed piles: a prospective randomized comparison with conventional haemorrhoidectomy. Colorectal Dis. 3:175–178.
7. Cheetham MJ, Cohen CR, Kamm MA, Phillips RK. (2003) A randomized, controlled trial of diathermy hemorrhoidectomy vs. stapled hemorrhoidectomy in an intended day-care setting with longer-term follow-up. Dis. Colon Rectum 46:491–497.
8. Chung CC, Cheung HY, Chan ES, Kwok SY, et al. (2005) Stapled hemorrhoidopexy vs. Harmonic Scalpel hemorrhoidectomy: a randomized trial. Dis. Colon Rectum 48:1213–1219.
9. Correa-Rovelo JM, Tellez O, Obregon L, Miranda-Gomez A, et al. (2002) Stapled rectal mucosectomy vs. closed hemorrhoidectomy: a randomized, clinical trial. Dis. Colon Rectum 45:1367–1374.
10. Ganio E, Altomare DF, Gabrielli F, Milito G, et al. (2001) Prospective randomized multicentre trial comparing stapled with open haemorrhoidectomy. Br. J. Surg. 88:669–674.
11. Helmy MA. (2000) Stapling procedure for hemorrhoids versus conventional haemorrhoidectomy. J. Egypt. Soc. Parasitol. 30:951–958.
12. Hetzer FH, Demartines N, Handschin AE, Clavien PA. (2002) Stapled vs excision hemorrhoidectomy: long-term results of a prospective randomized trial. Arch. Surg. 137:337–340.
13. Ho KS and Ho YH. (2006) Prospective randomized trial comparing stapled hemorrhoidopexy versus closed Ferguson hemorrhoidectomy. Tech. Coloproctol. 10:193–197.

14. Ho YH, Cheong WK, Tsang C, Ho J, et al. (2000) Stapled hemorrhoidectomy – cost and effectiveness. Randomized, controlled trial including incontinence scoring, anorectal manometry, and endoanal ultrasound assessments at up to three months. Dis. Colon Rectum 43:1666–1675.

15. Kairaluoma M, Nuorva K, Kellokumpu I. (2003) Day-case stapled (circular) vs. diathermy hemorrhoidectomy: a randomized, controlled trial evaluating surgical and functional outcome. Dis. Colon Rectum 46:93–99.

16. Kraemer M, Parulava T, Roblick M, Duschka L, et al. (2005) Prospective, randomized study: proximate PPH stapler vs. LigaSure for hemorrhoidal surgery. Dis. Colon Rectum 48:1517–1522.

17. Mehigan BJ, Monson JR, Hartley JE. (2000) Stapling procedure for haemorrhoids versus Milligan–Morgan haemorrhoidectomy: randomised controlled trial. Lancet 355:782–785.

18. Ortiz H, Marzo J, Armendariz P, de Miguel M. (2005) Stapled hemorrhoidopexy vs. diathermy excision for fourth-degree hemorrhoids: a randomized, clinical trial and review of the literature. Dis. Colon Rectum 48:809–815.

19. Palimento D, Picchio M, Attanasio U, Lombardi A, et al. (2003) Stapled and open hemorrhoidectomy: randomized controlled trial of early results. World J. Surg. 27:203–207.

20. Pavlidis T, Papaziogas B, Souparis A, Patsas A, et al. (2002) Modern stapled Longo procedure vs. conventional Milligan–Morgan hemorrhoidectomy: a randomized controlled trial. Int. J. Colorectal Dis. 17:50–53.

21. Racalbuto A, Aliotta I, Corsaro G, Lanteri R, et al. (2004) Hemorrhoidal stapler prolapsectomy vs. Milligan–Morgan hemorrhoidectomy: a long-term randomized trial. Int. J. Colorectal Dis. 19:239–244.

22. Rowsell M, Bello M, Hemingway DM. (2000) Circumferential mucosectomy (stapled haemorrhoidectomy) versus conventional haemorrhoidectomy: randomised controlled trial. Lancet 355:779–781.

23. Senagore AJ, Singer M, Abcarian H, Fleshman J, et al. (2004) A prospective, randomized, controlled multicenter trial comparing stapled hemorrhoidopexy and Ferguson hemorrhoidectomy: perioperative and one-year results. Dis. Colon Rectum 47:1824–1836.

24. Shalaby R and Desoky A. (2001) Randomized clinical trial of stapled versus Milligan–Morgan haemorrhoidectomy. Br. J. Surg. 88:1049–1053.

25. Smyth EF, Baker RP, Wilken BJ, Hartley JE, et al. (2003) Stapled versus excision haemorrhoidectomy: long-term follow up of a randomised controlled trial. Lancet 361:1437–1438.

26. Sutherland LM, Burchard AK, Matsuda K, Sweeney JL, et al. (2002) A systematic review of stapled hemorrhoidectomy. Arch. Surg. 137:1395–1406.

27. Wilson MS, Pope V, Doran HE, Fearn SJ, et al. (2002) Objective comparison of stapled anopexy and open hemorrhoidectomy: a randomized, controlled trial. Dis. Colon Rectum 45:1437–1444.

28. Ooi BS, Ho YH, Tang CL, Eu KW, et al. (2002) Results of stapling and conventional hemorrhoidectomy. Tech. Coloproctol. 6:59–60.

29. Picchio M, Palimento D, Attanasio U, Renda A. (2006) Stapled vs open hemorrhoidectomy: long-term outcome of a randomized controlled trial. Int. J. Colorectal Dis. 21:668–669.

30. Krska Z, Kvasnieka J, Faltyn J, Schmidt D, et al. (2003) Surgical treatment of haemorrhoids according to Longo and Milligan–Morgan: an evaluation of postoperative tissue response. Colorectal Dis. 5:573–576.

31. Lau PY, Meng WC, Yip AW. (2004) Stapled haemorrhoidectomy in Chinese patients: a prospective randomised control study. Hong Kong Med. J. 10:373–377.

32. Bikhchandani J, Agarwal PN, Kant R, Malik VK. (2005) Randomized controlled trial to compare the early and mid-term results of stapled versus open hemorrhoidectomy. Am. J. Surg. 189:56–60.

33. Basdanis G, Papadopoulos VN, Michalopoulos A, Apostolidis S, et al. (2005) Randomized clinical trial of stapled hemorrhoidectomy vs open with Ligasure for prolapsed piles. Surg. Endosc. 19:235–239.

34. Gravie JF, Lehur PA, Huten N, Papillon M, et al. (2005) Stapled hemorrhoidopexy versus Milligan–Morgan hemorrhoidectomy: a prospective, randomized, multicenter trial with 2-year postoperative follow up. Ann. Surg. 242:29–35.

35. Hasse C, Sitter H, Brune M, Wollenteit I, et al. (2004) [Haemorrhoidectomy: conventional excision versus resection with the circular stapler. Prospective, randomized study]. Dtsch. Med. Wochenschr. 129:1611–1617.

36. Ong CH, Chee Boon FE, Keng V. (2005) Ambulatory circular stapled haemorrhoidectomy under local anaesthesia versus circular stapled haemorrhoidectomy under regional anaesthesia. ANZ J. Surg. 75:184–186.

37. Schmidt MP, Fischbein J, Shatavi H. (2002) [Stapler hemorrhoidectomy versus conventional procedures – a clinical study]. Zentralbl. Chir. 127:15–18.

38. Johnson DB, DiSiena MR, Fanelli RD. (2003) Circumferential mucosectomy with stapled proctopexy is a safe, effective outpatient alternative for the treatment of symptomatic prolapsing hemorrhoids in the elderly. Surg. Endosc. 17:1990–1995.

39. Lomanto D and Katara AN. (2007) Stapled haemor-rhoidopexy for prolapsed haemorrhoids: short- and long-term experience. Asian J. Surg. 30:29–33.

40. Nahas SC, Borba MR, Brochado MC, Marques CF, et al. (2003) Stapled hemorrhoidectomy for the treatment of hemorrhoids. Arq. Gastroenterol. 40:35–39.

41. Morales-Olivera JM, Velasco L, Bada-Yllan O, Vergara-Fernandez O, et al. (2007) [First experience in surgical treatment of hemorrhoidal disease using the PPH stapler]. Rev. Invest. Clin. 59:108–111.

42. Ng KH, Eu KW, Ooi BS, Heah SM, et al. (2003) Stapled hemorrhoidopexy for prolapsed piles per-formed with concurrent perianal conditions. Tech. Coloproctol. 7:214–215.

43. Ng KH, Ho KS, Ooi BS, Tang CL, et al. (2006) Experience of 3711 stapled haemorrhoidectomy operations. Br. J. Surg. 93:226–230.

44. Ohana G, Myslovaty B, Ariche A, Dreznik Z, et al. (2007) Mid-term results of stapled hemorrhoidopexy for third- and fourth-degree hemorrhoids – correla-tion with the histological features of the resected tissue. World J. Surg. 31:1336–1342.

45. Papillon M, Arnaud JP, Descottes B, Gravie JF, et al. (1999) [Treatment of hemorrhoids with the Longo technique. Preliminary results of a prospective study on 94 cases]. Chirurgie 124:666–669.

46. Pernice LM, Bartalucci B, Bencini L, Borri A, et al. (2001) Early and late (ten years) experience with circular stapler hemorrhoidectomy. Dis. Colon Rectum 44:836–841.

47. Ravo B, Amato A, Bianco V, Boccasanta P, et al. (2002) Complications after stapled hemorrhoidectomy: can they be prevented? Tech. Coloproctol. 6:83–88.

48. Singer MA, Cintron JR, Fleshman JW, Chaudhry V, et al. (2002) Early experience with stapled hem-orrhoidectomy in the United States. Dis. Colon Rectum 45:360–367.

49. Slawik S, Kenefick N, Greenslade GL, Dixon AR. (2007) A prospective evaluation of stapled haemor-rhoidopexy/rectal mucosectomy in the management of 3rd and 4th degree haemorrhoids. Colorectal Dis. 9:352–356.

50. Sobrado CW, Cotti GC, Coelho FF, Rocha JR. (2006) Initial experience with stapled hemorrhoidopexy for treatment of hemorrhoids. Arq. Gastroenterol. 43:238–242.

51. Touzin E, Hegge S, McKinley C. (2006) Early expe-rience of stapled hemorrhoidectomy in a community hospital setting. Can. J. Surg. 49:316–320.

52. Trentin G, Agresta F, Mainente P, Ciardo L, et al. (2002) [Our experience in the treatment of hem-orrhoids and circumferential mucosal rectal prolapse using Longo muco-prolapsectomy]. Chir. Ital. 54: 389–394.

53. Varela GG and Castaneda Ortiz EM. (2006) [Hemorrhoidopexy with a PPH 03 circular sta-pler initial experience]. Rev. Gastroenterol. Mex. 71:288–295.

54. Abramowitz L, Godeberge P, Staumont G, Soudan D. (2001) Conference de consensus Traitment de la maladie hémorroïdaire. Ann. Chir. 126:845–849.

55. Corman ML, Gravie JF, Hager T, Loudon MA, et al. (2003) Stapled haemorrhoidopexy: a consensus position paper by an international working party – indications, contra-indications and technique. Colorectal Dis. 5:304–310.

56. Hemingway D. (2004) Stapled haemorrhoidectomy: a consensus paper. Colorectal Dis. 6:292

57. Warren BF. (2004) Stapled haemorrhoidectomy: a consensus paper. Colorectal Dis. 6:293

58. Lan P, Wu X, Zhou X, Wang J, et al. (2006) The safety and efficacy of stapled hemorrhoidectomy in the treatment of hemorrhoids: a systematic review and meta-analysis of ten randomized control trials. Int. J. Colorectal Dis. 21:172–178.

59. Nisar PJ, Acheson AG, Neal KR, Scholefield JH. (2004) Stapled hemorrhoidopexy compared with conventional hemorrhoidectomy: systematic review of randomized, controlled trials. Dis. Colon Rectum 47:1837–1845.

60. Silva JH. (2002) Pelvic lymphoscintigraphy: contri-bution to the preoperative staging of rectal cancer. Rev. Hosp. Clin. Fac. Med. Sao Paulo 57:55–62.

61. Tjandra JJ and Chan MK. (2007) Systematic review on the procedure for prolapse and hemorrhoids (sta-pled hemorrhoidopexy). Dis. Colon Rectum 50: 878–892.

62. Jayaraman S, Colquhoun PH, Malthaner RA. (2006) Stapled versus conventional surgery for hemor-rhoids. Cochrane Database Syst. Rev. CD005393

63. Lehur PA, Gravie JF, Meurette G. (2001) Circular stapled anopexy for haemorrhoidal disease: results. Colorectal Dis. 3:374–379.

64. Anghelacopoulos SE, Tagarakis GI, Pilpilidis I, Kartsounis C, et al. (2006) Albumin-glutaraldehyde bioadhesive ("Bioglue") for prevention of post-operative complications after stapled hemor-rhoidopexy: a randomized controlled trial. Wien. Klin. Wochenschr. 118:469–472.

65. Bozdag AD. (2005) A modified anoscope to facili-tate the purse-string suture for stapled hemor-rhoidopexy. Tech. Coloproctol. 9:239–242.

66. Carriero A, Dal Borgo P, Pucciani F. (2001) Stapled mucosal prolapsectomy for haemorrhoidal prolapse with Lone Star Retractor System. Tech. Coloproctol. 5:41–46.

67. Lloyd D, Ho KS, Seow-Choen F. (2002) Modified Longo's hemorrhoidectomy. Dis. Colon Rectum 45:416–417.

68. Regadas FS, Regadas SM, Rodrigues LV, Misici R, et al. (2005) New devices for stapled rectal mucosectomy: a multicenter experience. Tech. Coloproctol. 9:243–246.

69. Hoffman GH. (2006) Stapled hemorrhoidopexy: a new device and method of performance without using a pursestring suture. Dis. Colon Rectum 49:135–140.

70. Jayne DG and Seow-Choen F. (2002) Modified stapled haemorrhoidopexy for the treatment of massive circumferentially prolapsing piles. Tech. Coloproctol. 6:191–193.

71. Beck J and Szinicz G. (2001) Modified technique of stapled hemorroidectomy. Acta Chir. Austriaca 189:56–60.

72. Aumann G, Petersen S, Pollack T, Hellmich G, et al. (2004) Severe intra-abdominal bleeding following stapled mucosectomy due to enterocele: report of a case. Tech. Coloproctol. 8:41–43.

73. Blouhos K, Vasiliadis K, Tsalis K, Botsios D, et al. (2007) Uncontrollable intra-abdominal bleeding necessitating low anterior resection of the rectum after stapled hemorrhoidopexy: report of a case. Surg. Today 37:254–257.

74. Bonner C, Prohm P, Storkel S. (2001) [Fournier gangrene as a rare complication after stapler hemorrhoidectomy. Case report and review of the literature]. Chirurg 72:1464–1466.

75. Brusciano L, Ayabaca SM, Pescatori M, Accarpio GM, et al. (2004) Reinterventions after complicated or failed stapled hemorrhoidopexy. Dis. Colon Rectum 47:1846–1851.

76. Cheetham MJ, Mortensen NJ, Nystrom PO, Kamm MA, et al. (2000) Persistent pain and faecal urgency after stapled haemorrhoidectomy. Lancet 356:730–733.

77. Filingeri V and Gravante G. (2005) Pneumoretroperitoneum, pneumomediastinum and subcutaneous emphysema of the neck after stapled hemorrhoidopexy. Tech. Coloproctol. 9:86

78. Giebel GD. (2002) [Comment on Ch. Bonner et al.: Fournier gangrene as a rare complication after stapler hemorrhoidectomy]. Chirurg 73:288

79. Herold A and Kirsch JJ. (2000) Pain after stapled haemorrhoidectomy. Lancet 356:2187

80. Ho YH, Seow-Choen F, Tsang C, Eu KW. (2001) Randomized trial assessing anal sphincter injuries after stapled haemorrhoidectomy. Br. J. Surg. 88:1449–1455.

81. Huang WS, Chin CC, Yeh CH, Lin PY, et al. (2007) The late onset of an anal abscess caused by a chicken bone that complicated stapled hemorrhoidopexy. Int. J. Colorectal Dis. 22:1291–1292

82. Jongen J, Bock JU, Peleikis HG, Eberstein A, et al. (2006) Complications and reoperations in stapled anopexy: learning by doing. Int. J. Colorectal Dis. 21:166–171.

83. Kanellos I, Blouhos K, Demetriades H, Pramateftakis MG, et al. (2004) Pneumomediastinum after dilatation of anal stricture following stapled hemorrhoidopexy. Tech. Coloproctol. 8:185–187.

84. Maw A, Eu KW, Seow-Choen F. (2002) Retroperitoneal sepsis complicating stapled hemorrhoidectomy: report of a case and review of the literature. Dis. Colon Rectum 45:826–828.

85. Molloy RG and Kingsmore D. (2000) Life threatening pelvic sepsis after stapled haemorrhoidectomy. Lancet 355:810

86. Pescatori M. (2000) Pain after stapled haemorrhoidectomy. Lancet 356:2188

87. Pescatori M, Spyrou M, Cobellis L, Bottini C, et al. (2006) The rectal pocket syndrome after stapled mucosectomy. Colorectal Dis. 8:808–811.

88. Petersen S, Hellmich G, Schumann D, Schuster A, et al. (2004) Early rectal stenosis following stapled rectal mucosectomy for hemorrhoids. BMC Surg. 4:6

89. Ripetti V, Caricato M, Arullani A. (2002) Rectal perforation, retropneumoperitoneum, and pneumomediastinum after stapling procedure for prolapsed hemorrhoids: report of a case and subsequent considerations. Dis. Colon Rectum 45:268–270.

90. Roos P. (2000) Haemorrhoid surgery revised. Lancet 355:1648

91. Wong LY, Jiang JK, Chang SC, Lin JK. (2003) Rectal perforation: a life-threatening complication of stapled hemorrhoidectomy: report of a case. Dis. Colon Rectum 46:116–117.

92. Yao L, Zhong Y, Xu J, Xu M, et al. (2006) Rectal stenosis after procedures for prolapse and hemorrhoids (PPH) – a report from China. World J. Surg. 30:1311–1315.

93. Herold A, Kirsch J, Staude G, Hager T, et al. (2000) A German multicentre study on circular stapled haemorrhoidectomy. Colorectal Dis. 2(Suppl):18

94. Oughriss M, Yver R, Faucheron JL. (2005) Complications of stapled hemorrhoidectomy: a French multicentric study. Gastroenterol. Clin. Biol. 29:429–433.

95. Pessaux P, Tuech JJ, Laurent B, Regenet N, et al. (2004) [Morbidity after stapled haemorrhoidectomy: long-term results about 140 patients and review of the literature]. Ann. Chir. 129:571–577.

96. Correa-Rovelo JM, Tellez O, Obregon L, Duque-Lopez X, et al. (2003) Prospective study of factors affecting postoperative pain and symptom persistence after stapled rectal mucosectomy for hemorrhoids: a need for preservation of squamous epithelium. Dis. Colon Rectum 46:955–962.

97. Pigot F, Dao-Quang M, Castinel A, Juguet F, et al. (2006) Low hemorrhoidopexy staple line does not

improve results and increases risk for incontinence. Tech. Coloproctol. 10:329–333.

98. Plocek MD, Kondylis LA, Duhan-Floyd N, Reilly JC, et al. (2006) Hemorrhoidopexy staple line height predicts return to work. Dis. Colon Rectum 49:1905–1909.

99. Mlakar B and Kosorok P. (2005) Flavonoids to reduce bleeding and pain after stapled hemorrhoidopexy: a randomized controlled trial. Wien. Klin. Wochenschr. 117:558–560.

100. Koh DC, Cheong DM, Wong KS. (2005) Stapled haemorrhoidectomy: bothersome staple line bleeding. Asian J. Surg. 28:193–197.

101. Ganio E, Altomare DF, Milito G, Gabrielli F, et al. (2007) Long-term outcome of a multicentre randomized clinical trial of stapled haemorrhoidopexy versus Milligan–Morgan haemorrhoidectomy. Br. J. Surg. 94:1033–1037.

102. Ortiz H, Marzo J, Armendariz P. (2002) Randomized clinical trial of stapled haemorrhoidopexy versus conventional diathermy haemorrhoidectomy. Br. J. Surg. 89:1376–1381.

103. Peng BC, Jayne DG, Ho YH. (2003) Randomized trial of rubber band ligation vs. stapled hemorrhoidectomy for prolapsed piles. Dis. Colon Rectum 46:291–297.

104. Van de SJ, D'Hoore A, Duinslaeger M, Chasse E, et al. (2005) Long-term results after excision haemorrhoidectomy versus stapled haemorrhoidopexy for prolapsing haemorrhoids; a Belgian prospective randomized trial. Acta Chir. Belg. 105:44–52.

105. Mattana C, Coco C, Manno A, Verbo A, et al. (2007) Stapled hemorrhoidopexy and Milligan–Morgan hemorrhoidectomy in the cure of fourth-degree hemorrhoids: long-term evaluation and clinical results. Dis. Colon Rectum 50:1770–1775.

106. Cook T, Guyatt GH, Laupacis A, Sackett DL, et al. (1992) Rules of evidence and clinical recommendation on the use of antithrombotic agents. Chest 102:305S–311S.

107. Sackett DL. (1989) Rules of evidence and clinical recommendations on the use of antithrombotic agents. Chest 95:2S–4S.

108. Zacharakis E, Kanellos D, Pramateftakis MG, Kanellos I, et al. (2007) Long-term results after stapled haemorrhoidopexy for fourth-degree haemorrhoids: a prospective study with median follow-up of 6 years. Tech. Coloproctol. 11:144–147.

109. Parvaiz A, Azeem S, Singh RK, Lamparelli M. (2006) Stapled hemorrhoidopexy: an alternative technique for the treatment of bleeding anorectal varices. Report of a case. Dis. Colon Rectum 49:411–412.

110. Biswas S, George ML, Leather AJ. (2003) Stapled anopexy in the treatment of anal varices: report of a case. Dis. Colon Rectum 46:1284–1285.

111. Huang WS, Lin PY, Chin CC, Yeh CH, et al. (2007) Stapled hemorrhoidopexy for prolapsed hemorrhoids in patients with liver cirrhosis; a preliminary outcome for 8-case experience. Int. J. Colorectal Dis. 22:1083–1089

112. Fantin AC, Hetzer FH, Christ AD, Fried M, et al. (2002) Influence of stapler haemorrhoidectomy on anorectal function and on patients' acceptance. Swiss. Med. Wkly 132:38–42.

113. Lunniss PJ, Gladman MA, Hetzer FH, Williams NS, et al. (2004) Risk factors in acquired faecal incontinence. J. R. Soc. Med. 97:111–116.

114. Mlakar B. (2007) Should we avoid stapled hemorrhoidopexy in males and females who practice receptive anal sex? Dis. Colon Rectum 50:1727

115. Kekez T, Bulic K, Smudj D, Majerovic M. (2007) Is stapled hemorrhoidopexy safe for the male homosexual patient? Report of a case. Surg. Today 37:335–337.

116. Guy RJ, Ng CE, Eu KW. (2003) Stapled anoplasty for haemorrhoids: a comparison of ambulatory vs. in-patient procedures. Colorectal Dis. 5:29–32.

117. Beattie GC, McAdam TK, McIntosh SA, Loudon MA. (2006) Day case stapled haemorrhoidopexy for prolapsing haemorrhoids. Colorectal Dis. 8:56–61.

118. Gabrielli F, Chiarelli M, Cioffi U, Guttadauro A, et al. (2001) Day surgery for mucosal-hemorrhoidal prolapse using a circular stapler and modified regional anesthesia. Dis. Colon Rectum 44:842–844.

119. Mariani P, Arrigoni G, Quartierini G, Dapri G, et al. (2005) Local anesthesia for stapled prolapsectomy in day surgery: results of a prospective trial. Dis. Colon Rectum 48:1447–1450.

120. Kirsch JJ, Staude G, Herold A. (2001) [The Longo and Milligan–Morgan hemorrhoidectomy. A prospective comparative study of 300 patients]. Chirurg 72:180–185.

121. Martinsons A, Narbuts Z, Brunenieks I, Pavars M, et al. (2007) A comparison of quality of life and postoperative results from combined PPH and conventional haemorrhoidectomy in different cases of haemorrhoidal disease. Colorectal Dis. 9:423–429.

122. Fueglistaler P, Guenin MO, Montali I, Kern B, et al. (2007) Long-term results after stapled hemorrhoidopexy: high patient satisfaction despite frequent postoperative symptoms. Dis. Colon Rectum 50:204–212.

123. Delikoukos S, Zacharoulis D, Hatzitheofilou C. (2005) Stapled hemorrhoidectomy under local

anesthesia: tips and tricks. Dis. Colon Rectum 48:2153–2155.

124. Esser S, Khubchandani I, Rakhmanine M. (2004) Stapled hemorrhoidectomy with local anesthesia can be performed safely and cost-efficiently. Dis. Colon Rectum 47:1164–1169.

125. Gerjy R, Derwinger K, Nystrom PO. (2006) Perianal local block for stapled anopexy. Dis. Colon Rectum 49:1914–1921.

126. Maw A, Concepcion R, Eu KW, Seow-Choen F, et al. (2003) Prospective randomized study of bacteraemia in diathermy and stapled haemorrhoidectomy. Br. J. Surg. 90:222–226.

127. Goulimaris I, Kanellos I, Christoforidis E, Mantzoros I, et al. (2002) Stapled haemorrhoidectomy compared with Milligan–Morgan excision for the treatment of prolapsing haemorrhoids: a prospective study. Eur. J. Surg. 168:621–625.

128. Colak T, Akca T, Dirlik M, Kanik A, et al. (2003) Micronized flavonoids in pain control after hemorrhoidectomy: a prospective randomized controlled study. Surg. Today 33:828–832.

129. Ho YH and Seow-Choen F. (2000) Randomized clinical trial of micronized flavonoids in the early control of bleeding from acute internal haemorrhoids. Br. J. Surg. 87:1732–1733.

130. La Torre F and Nicolai AP. (2004) Clinical use of micronized purified flavonoid fraction for treatment of symptoms after hemorrhoidectomy: results of a randomized, controlled, clinical trial. Dis. Colon Rectum 47:704–710.

131. Perez-Vicente F, Arroyo A, Serrano P, Candela F, et al. (2006) Prospective randomised clinical trial of single versus double purse-string stapled mucosectomy in the treatment of prolapsed haemorrhoids. Int. J. Colorectal Dis. 21:38–43.

132. Arroyo A, Perez-Vicente F, Miranda E, Sanchez A, et al. (2006) Prospective randomized clinical trial comparing two different circular staplers for mucosectomy in the treatment of hemorrhoids. World J. Surg. 30:1305–1310.

133. Angelone G, Giardiello C, Prota C. (2007) Bleeding after stapled haemorrhoidopexy using the PPH 03 stapler device. Experience and results in 100 consecutive patients. Chir. Ital. 59:225–229.

134. Lim YK, Eu KW, Ho KS, Ooi BS, et al. (2006) PPH03 stapled hemorrhoidopexy: our experience. Tech. Coloproctol. 10:43–46.

135. Khalil KH, O'Bichere A, Sellu D. (2000) Randomized clinical trial of sutured versus stapled closed haemorrhoidectomy. Br. J. Surg. 87:1352–1355.

136. Zmora O, Colquhoun P, Abramson S, Weiss EG, et al. (2004) Can the procedure for prolapsing hemorrhoids (PPH) be done twice? Results of a porcine model. Surg. Endosc. 18:757–761.

137. Yamamoto J, Nagai M, Smith TB, Tamaki S, et al. (2006) Adaptation of the pursestring suture anoscope with a small hole in a case of stapled hemorrhoidectomy. Dis. Colon Rectum 49:925–926.

138. Guenin MO, Kern B, Ackermann C. (2005) Modification of the dilator used for Longo hemorrhoidectomy]. J. Chir. (Paris) 142:406

139. Mathur P, Ho T, Spalinger R, Chirurgie FM, et al. (2004) The "winged" circular anal dilator in stapled hemorrhoidectomy. Dis. Colon Rectum 47:542–543.

140. Forshaw MJ, Mhandu PC, Parker MC. (2005) The use of the Deaver retractor to visualize staple line haemorrhage following stapled anopexy. Colorectal Dis. 7:96–97.

141. Altomare DF, Rinaldi M, Sallustio PL, Martino P, et al. (2001) Long-term effects of stapled haemorrhoidectomy on internal anal function and sensitivity. Br. J. Surg. 88:1487–1491.

142. Shanmugam V, Watson AJ, Chapman AD, Binnie NR, et al. (2005) Pathological audit of stapled haemorrhoidopexy. Colorectal Dis. 7:172–175.

143. Weyand G, Webels F, Celebi H, Ommer A, et al. (2002) [Anal pressures after stapler hemorrhoidectomy – a prospective analysis of 33 patients]. Zentralbl. Chir. 127:22–24.

144. Gravie JF. (2002) [The Longo technique: should it be adopted?]. Ann. Chir. 127:327–329.

145. Boccasanta P, Venturi M, Roviaro G. (2007) Stapled transanal rectal resection versus stapled anopexy in the cure of hemorrhoids associated with rectal prolapse. A randomized controlled trial. Int. J. Colorectal Dis. 22:245–251.

146. Angelone G, Giardiello C, Prota C. (2006) Stapled hemorrhoidopexy. Complications and 2-year follow-up. Chir. Ital. 58:753–760.

147. McDonald PJ, Bona R, Cohen CR. (2004) Rectovaginal fistula after stapled haemorrhoidopexy. Colorectal Dis. 6:64–65.

148. Kohlstadt CM, Weber J, Prohm P. (1999) Die Stapler-Hämorrhoidektomie-Eine neue Alternative zu den konventionellen Methoden. Zentralbl. Chir. 124:238–243.

149. Arnaud JP, Pessaux P, Huten N, De Manzini N, et al. (2001) Treatment of hemorrhoids with circular stapler, a new alternative to conventional methods: a prospective study of 140 patients. J. Am. Coll. Surg. 193:161–165.

150. Stukavec J and Horak L. (2006) [Complications of the Longo Procedure – rectal occlusion]. Rozhl. Chir. 85:517–519.

151. Rowsell M, Bello M, Hemingway DM. (2000) Pain after stapled haemorrhoidectomy. Lancet 356:2188

152. Seow-Choen F. (2001) Stapled haemorrhoidectomy: pain or gain. Br. J. Surg. 88:1–3.

153. Wexner SD. (2001) Persistent pain and faecal urgency after stapled haemorrhoidectomy. Tech. Coloproctol. 5:56–57.

154. Williams R, Kondylis L, Geisler D, Kondylis P. (2007) Stapled hemorrhoidopexy height as outcome indicator. Am. J. Surg. 193:336–339.

155. Bufo A, Galasse S, Amoroso M. (2006) Recurrent severe postoperative bleeding after stapled hemorrhoidopexy requiring emergency laparotomy. Tech. Coloproctol. 10:62–63.

156. Grau LA, Budo AH, Fantova MJ, Sala XS. (2005) Perirectal haematoma and hypovolaemic shock after rectal stapled mucosectomy for haemorrhoids. Int. J. Colorectal Dis. 20:471–472.

157. Cotton MH. (2005) Pelvic sepsis after stapled hemorrhoidectomy. J. Am. Coll. Surg. 200:983

158. Daniel F, Sultan S, de Parades V, Bauer P, et al. (2006) Anal fissure and minor anorectal sepsis after stapled hemorrhoidectomy. Dis. Colon Rectum 49:693–694.

159. McCloud JM, Doucas H, Scott AD, Jameson JS. (2007) Delayed presentation of life-threatening perineal sepsis following stapled haemorrhoidectomy: a case report. Ann. R. Coll. Surg. Engl. 89:301–302.

160. Pessaux P, Lermite E, Tuech JJ, Brehant O, et al. (2004) Pelvic sepsis after stapled hemorrhoidectomy. J. Am. Coll. Surg. 199:824–825.

161. Ravo B. (2005) Septic complications after stapled hemorrhoidectomy. J. Am. Coll. Surg. 201:155–156.

162. NICE. (2007) Technology Appraisal Guidance 128: stapled haemorrhoidopexy for the treatment of haemorrhoids. Available at http://www.nice.org.uk/TA128.

163. Farinetti A and Saviano M. (2000) [Surgical treatment of hemorrhoidal disease using circular mechanical stapler. Analysis of costs]. Minerva Chir. 55:401–407.

164. Longo A. (2003) Obstructed defecation because of rectal pathologies. Novel surgical treatment: stapled transanal resection (STARR). Proceedings of the 14th Annual International Colorectal Disease Symposium, Ft Lauderdale, FL, February 13–15.

165. Agachan F, Chen T, Pfeifer J, Reissman P, et al. (1996) A constipation scoring system to simplify evaluation and management of constipated patients. Dis. Colon Rectum 39:681–685.

166. Dodi G, Pietroletti R, Milito G, Binda G, et al. (2003) Bleeding, incontinence, pain and constipation after STARR transanal double stapling rectotomy for obstructed defecation. Tech. Coloproctol. 7:148–153.

167. Boccasanta P, Venturi M, Stuto A, Bottini C, et al. (2004) Stapled transanal rectal resection for outlet obstruction: a prospective, multicenter trial. Dis. Colon Rectum 47:1285–1296.

168. Boccasanta P, Venturi M, Salamina G, Cesana BM, et al. (2004) New trends in the surgical treatment of outlet obstruction: clinical and functional results of two novel transanal stapled techniques from a randomised controlled trial. Int. J. Colorectal Dis. 19:359–369.

169. Schwandner O, Farke S, Bruch HP. (2005) Stapled transanal rectal resection (STARR) for obstructed defection caused by rectocele and rectoanal intussusception. Viszeralchirurgie 40:331–41.

170. Ommer A, Albrecht K, Wenger F, Walz MK. (2006) Stapled transanal rectal resection (STARR): a new option in the treatment of obstructive defecation syndrome. Langenbecks Arch. Surg. 391:32–37.

171. Ommer A, Köhler A, Athana S, Athanasiadis S. (1998) Ergebnisse der transperinealen Levatorplastik bei der Behandlung de symptomatischen Rektocele. Chirurg 69:966–972.

172. Renzi A, Izzo D, Di Sarno G, Izzo G, et al. (2006) Stapled transanal rectal resection to treat obstructed defecation caused by rectal intussusception and rectocele. Int. J. Colorectal Dis. 21:661–667.

173. Sielaff M, Scherer R, Gögler H, Farke S. (2006) Die STARR-Operation. Coloproctology 28: 217–223.

174. Arroyo A, Perez-Vicente F, Serrano P, Sanchez A, et al. (2007) Evaluation of the stapled transanal rectal resection technique with two staplers in the treatment of obstructive defecation syndrome. J. Am. Coll. Surg. 204:56–63.

175. Pechlivanides G, Tsiaoussis J, Athanasakis E, Zervakis N, et al. (2007) Stapled transanal rectal resection (STARR) to reverse the anatomic disorders of pelvic floor dyssynergia. World J. Surg. 31:1329–1335.

176. Boccasanta P, Venturi M, Calabro G, Maciocco M, et al. (2008) Stapled transanal rectal resection in solitary rectal ulcer associated with prolapse of the rectum: a prospective study. Dis. Colon Rectum 51:348–354.

177. Gagliardi G, Pescatori M, Altomare DF, Binda GA, et al. (2008) Results, outcome predictors, and complications after stapled transanal rectal resection for obstructed defecation. Dis. Colon Rectum 51:186–195.

178. Frascio M, Stabilini C, Ricci B, Marino P, et al. (2008) Stapled transanal rectal resection for outlet obstruction syndrome: results and follow-up. World J. Surg. 32:1110–5.

179. NICE. (2007) Interventional Procedure Guidance 169: Stapled transanal rectal resection for obstructed

dcfaccation syndrome. Available at http://www.nice.org.uk/IPG169.

180. Pescatori M, Favetta D, Dedola S, Orsini S. (1997) Transanal stapled excision of rectal mucosal prolapse. Tech. Coloproctol. 1:96–98.

181. Altomare DF, Rinaldi M, Veglia A, Petrolino M, et al. (2002) Combined perineal and endorectal repair of rectocele by circular stapler: a novel surgical technique. Dis. Colon Rectum 45:1549–1552.

182. Corman ML, Carriero A, Hager T, Herold A, et al. (2006) Consensus conference on the stapled transanal rectal resection (STARR) for disordered defaecation. Colorectal Dis. 8:98–101.

183. Petersen S, Hellmich G, Schuster A, Lehmann D, et al. (2006) Stapled transanal rectal resection under laparoscopic surveillance for rectocele and concomitant enterocele. Dis. Colon Rectum 49:685–689.

184. Sciaudone G, Di Stazio C, Guadagni I, Selvaggi F. (2007) Rectal diverticulum: a new complication of STARR procedure for obstructed defecation. Tech. Coloproctol. 12:61–3.

185. Bassi R, Rademacher J, Savoia A. (2006) Rectovaginal fistula after STARR procedure complicated by haematoma of the posterior vaginal wall: report of a case. Tech. Coloproctol. 10:361–363.

186. Li DG, Scilletta B, Tomaselli TG, Zarbo G. (2008) Rectovaginal fistula: a new approach by stapled transanal rectal resection. J. Gastrointest. Surg. 12:601–603.

Chapter 9
Areas of Controversy and Future Research

D.G. Jayne and A. Stuto

Introduction

It is now almost 10 years since Antonio Longo presented his paper on transanal stapling for hemorrhoidal prolapse to the World Congress of Endoscopic Surgery in Rome in 1998 [1]. In that time our understanding of the pathophysiology underlying hemorrhoidal prolapse and obstructed defecation syndrome has advanced.

Experience with transanal stapling for these conditions has shown it to be safe and effective, at least in the short term. Methods have evolved in an attempt to eliminate complications and improve results, and the concept of transanal stapling has been extended to full-thickness rectal resection (STARR procedure) for the treatment of internal rectal prolapse associated with obstructed defecation. Originally, this was performed as a double-stapling procedure utilizing the PPH-01™ instrument, but more recently a stapler specifically designed for STARR, the Contour30™, has been introduced.

Despite the initial success and the subsequent advances in transanal stapling for anorectal prolapse, there remains many areas of uncertainty and controversy. The aim of this chapter is to explore these areas, to identify gaps in our knowledge, and to suggest possible avenues for future research.

Stapled Hemorrhoidopexy

The incorporation of stapled hemorrhoidopexy into routine surgical practice has been slow, with sporadic uptake by enthusiasts and outright rejection by others. Initial enthusiasm, at least in the United Kingdom, was fueled by two small randomized trials reporting good short-term safety and efficacy compared to Milligan–Morgan hemorrhoidectomy [2, 3]. However, this was quickly followed by concern provoked by the reporting of persistent anorectal pain and defecatory urgency [4, 5] and the possibility of life-threatening perianal sepsis [6]. These concerns had a negative influence on the uptake of stapled hemorrhoidopexy until encouraging results from individual series and randomized trials began to appear [7–15]. This was followed by a renewed confidence in the procedure and a gradual acceptance that stapled hemorrhoidopexy had a place in the modern management of hemorrhoidal disease. Currently, although stapled hemorrhoidopexy is accepted as a method for dealing with symptomatic prolapsing piles, it is still not universally regarded as the preferred first-line treatment option. Some of the reasons for this are discussed later. The literature contains many individual series, randomized trials, and meta-analyses reporting the outcomes of stapled hemorrhoidopexy (see Chap. 8).The majority of these studies have concentrated on short-term outcomes of safety and efficacy and have shown a benefit for stapled hemorrhoidopexy in terms of reduced postoperative pain and earlier return to normal function. However, many of these studies consist of relatively small patient numbers and differences in study design, and the outcomes measured make comparison and clinical interpretation difficult.

D. Jayne and A. Stuto (eds.), Transanal Stapling Techniques for Anorectal Prolapse,
DOI: 10.1007/978-1-84800-905-9_9, © Springer-Verlag London Limited 2009

The Current Status of Stapled Hemorrhoidopexy

The current status of stapled hemorrhoidopexy is probably best summarized in the National Institute for Health and Clinical Excellence (NICE) guidelines published in September 2007 [16]. These recommendations were based on a meta-analysis undertaken by the Health Economics Unit at the University of York, UK. The meta-analysis included 27 randomized controlled trials and a total of 2,279 patients. The analysis only considered stapled hemorrhoidopexy performed by the single-stapled PPH-01™ technique and compared it to conventional hemorrhoidectomy (Milligan–Morgan, Ferguson, or their derivatives). Many of the short-term outcomes could not be subjected to statistical analysis due to data heterogeneity, but better outcomes were observed following stapled hemorrhoidopexy with reduced operating times, shorter hospital stay, and quicker return to normal activity. A significant reduction in postoperative pain was observed following stapled hemorrhoidopexy. The numbers of patients reporting long-term pain was low after both stapled hemorrhoidopexy and conventional hemorrhoidectomy with no difference between the two. Previous meta-analyses had suggested that the incidence of early postoperative bleeding was reduced following stapled hemorrhoidopexy [17, 18], but analysis of the more mature data in the 2007 NICE review failed to show a difference in either the early- or long-term rates of bleeding between the two techniques. As one might expect, one of the main benefits of stapled hemorrhoidopexy was a significant reduction in postoperative wound complications. All trials reporting on wound healing recorded complete wound healing by 12 weeks after stapled hemorrhoidopexy, as compared to continuing problems in 6–20% of conventional hemorrhoidectomy wounds. Importantly, the rates of postoperative complications were similar after both stapled hemorrhoidopexy and conventional hemorrhoidectomy. The much-feared complications of perianal fistulation, sepsis, and fecal incontinence were rare after both procedures.

In the short term, therefore, evidence would suggest that stapled hemorrhoidopexy is at least as safe as conventional hemorrhoidectomy, with benefits in terms of short-term recovery. The controversy emerges when one looks at the long-term outcomes, particularly in respect to the incidence of recurrent prolapse. Several authors have reported an increased rate of recurrent prolapse following stapled hemorrhoidectomy with an incidence ranging from 2 to 24% [19–26]. This is seldom seen after conventional hemorrhoidectomy [27]. The increased recurrent prolapse rate after stapled hemorrhoidopexy was confirmed in the NICE 2007 analysis, with patients followed for greater than 12 months having a 4.34-fold greater risk (odds ratio: 4.34, 95%CI: 1.67, 11.28; $p = 0.003$). This was mirrored by an increased reintervention rate for recurrent prolapse (odds ratio: 5.78; 95%CI: 2.0, 23.0, $p = 0.002$).

Naturally, this raises questions as to the cause of recurrent prolapse following stapled hemorrhoidopexy. Is it due to poor surgical technique, a deficiency in the stapling technology, or related to disease severity and patient selection? It has been suggested that recurrent prolapse may be related to the volume of hemorrhoidal tissue to be excised, and this is supported by a higher recurrence rate in patients undergoing stapled hemorrhoidopexy for grade IV as compared to grade III hemorrhoidal disease [20]. The issue of recurrent prolapse and strategies to prevent its occurrence are discussed in more detail later.

Until overwhelming evidence in favor of stapled hemorrhoidopexy is forthcoming, it is likely that surgical opinion will remain divided and that uptake of the stapling procedure will continue to be determined by surgeon preference. Similar to other areas of technological development, it is likely that with the passage of time patient preference will also come to influence decision making. This is particularly so as patient awareness concerning medical treatment increases with ready access to health care information via the internet. An array of techniques is now available for the treatment of prolapsing piles, and it is likely that further techniques and modifications will emerge. When deciding which treatment is preferred, the patient is faced with a confounding array of options. If he is advised that excisional surgery is needed, which of the available techniques should he choose? Should he opt for conventional hemorrhoidectomy either by the Milligan–Morgan or Ferguson technique or one of the newer modifications incorporating

Ligasure or Ultrasonic dissection? Alternatively he could choose stapled hemorrhoidopexy or the less-invasive Hemorrhoidal Artery Ligation System (HALS). This is an almost impossible decision for the majority of patients, who are likely to put their trust in their clinician to advise them appropriately. Unfortunately randomized trials comparing stapled hemorrhoidopexy with techniques other than Milligan–Morgan hemorrhoidectomy are limited. Peng et al. compared the use of rubber-band ligation with stapled hemorrhoidopexy for grade III and small grade IV hemorrhoidal prolapse [28]. As expected, stapled hemorrhoidopexy was associated with increased postintervention pain and narcotic usage. Although both techniques produced similar control of symptomatic prolapse, the rate of recurrent bleeding was greater following rubber-band ligation. The authors concluded that although the minor complication rate was higher after stapled hemorrhoidopexy, it offered the best chance of a "one-off" symptomatic cure. Further research comparing stapled hemorrhoidopexy with other treatment modalities is required to facilitate patient information and surgical decision making.

Controversies in Surgical Technique

Despite initial concerns regarding intractable post-operative pain and defecatory urgency [4, 5], it is reassuring that the overall reported incidence of these complications is low. It would appear that many of these complications occurred early in the experience of stapled hemorrhoidopexy and were likely a consequence of the learning curve associated with the new technology. The placement of a staple line in close proximity to the dentate line, at or on the sensitive anoderm, will inevitably result in anorectal pain and urgency which will persist until such time as the irritant stimulus is been removed, and complete re-epithelialization of the anastomosis has occurred.

With experience we have learnt the fundamental principles that must be observed to ensure a satisfactory result with low morbidity. Care must be observed in the placement of the anal retractor to avoid rapid sphincter dilatation and internal sphincter fragmentation, which will result in passive fecal soiling. The purse-string suture should be placed well above the dentate line, at or above the apex

of the hemorrhoidal pedicles, with the aims of the procedure kept in mind. These are threefold (a) to remove excess hemorrhoidal tissue, (b) to restore and fix the prolapsed hemorrhoidal tissue back in its normal anatomical position, and (c) to reduce hemorrhoidal vascularity by interruption of the submucosal vascular supply. It is not the aim of the procedure to remove the hemorrhoidal tissue in its entirety. Such a maneuver will invariably result in a low staple line, causing pain and urgency. Rather, it should be aimed to leave the lower hemorrhoidal tissue that supports the transitional epithelium of the anal canal and is involved in the rectoanal inhibitory reflex, anal sampling and the control of normal continence.

Previous work has attempted to determine the ideal height of the staple line in order to avoid unnecessary postoperative pain. In a pathological study of 106 stapled hemorrhoidopexy specimens, no correlation was observed between the presence of squamous epithelium in the resection specimen and symptomatic outcomes or postoperative continence [29]. However, this study only included 19 resection specimens in which squamous epithelium was present, and clinical outcomes were assessed by postal questionnaire rather than patient interview and examination. A study by Plocek et al. utilizing a prospective database of 75 patients undergoing stapled hemorrhoidopexy suggested that a staple line > 22 mm above the dentate line was associated with a reduced need for postoperative narcotics and an earlier return to work [30]. This was corroborated by Williams et al. who found that patients with a staple line > 20 mm above the dentate line had a shorter use of postoperative narcotics, whereas analgesic usage was prolonged in patients with squamous epithelium present in the resection specimen [31]. However, if the staple line exceeded 40 mm above the dentate line poorer outcomes in terms of symptom recurrence were observed.

It is the authors' opinion that the use of the dentate line as a reference point should be discouraged as it is seldom visible as a discrete operative landmark when effaced by the dilating anal retractor. Rather, the anorectal junction, palpable at the top of the puborectalis sling posteriorly, and the apices of the hemorrhoidal pedicles are to be preferred. Although a staple line of > 20 mm above the dentate line may be useful as a rough guide, it should be borne in mind that the length of the anal canal varies considerably with patient sex and build, such that a staple line height of 20 mm in a well-built male may well impinge on the dentate line. Consideration should also be given to the fact that the height of placement of the purse-string suture does not necessarily dictate the height of the resultant stapled anastomosis. The guiding principle, however, is that the height of the mucosal resection should be such that it avoids placement of the staple line in proximity to the sensitive anoderm, while not being so high that the resection is in essence a rectal mucosal biopsy which will not achieve the desired hemorrhoidal excision. Accurate placement of the purse-string suture, to achieve adequate hemorrhoidal resection while avoiding encroachment on the dentate line, is perhaps the most challenging aspect of stapled hemorrhoidopexy and is often only learnt through experience.

One of the advantages of stapled hemorrhoidopexy in terms of operative intervention appears to be a similar [16] or even reduced rate [21, 24] of early postoperative bleeding when compared to conventional hemorrhoidectomy. However, most of the data are derived from studies utilizing the PPH01 stapler. Few studies have compared the effect of the reduced staple height in the newer PPH03 device with that of the original PPH01 stapler and have reported a benefit not just in terms of postoperative bleeding but also patient-reported discomfort on defecation [32]. This was attributed to the less frequent occurrence of granulomas at the site of the staple line following PPH03 hemorrhoidopexy.

The reduced postoperative pain associated with stapled hemorrhoidopexy makes it attractive as a day-case procedure using either general or regional anesthesia [33, 34]. In addition, the shorter hospital stay and earlier return to work may offset the cost of the stapling device [8, 35]. The antagonists of stapled hemorrhoidopexy, however, would argue that Milligan–Morgan hemorrhoidectomy can also be performed effectively as a day-case procedure with acceptable levels of patient discomfort. With adequate postoperative care, it is claimed that previously quoted hospital stays of 3–5 days following conventional hemorrhoidectomy can be reduced to that comparable to stapled hemorrhoidopexy, and if outcomes are equivalent then the additional cost of the stapling gun cannot be justified. When interpreting the evidence it should be borne in mind that it is relatively easy to discharge a patient home on the day of surgery, provided that sufficient local anesthetic and postoperative analgesia has been administered. However, it is once the patient is home and the local anesthetic effect has worn off that the patient experiences maximal pain. Pain in the first week after surgery is therefore probably the true indicator of postoperative discomfort, rather than that experience immediately after surgery and prior to discharge.

Although the majority of patients undergoing stapled hemorrhoidopexy will experience an acceptable degree of postoperative discomfort, there remains a minority for whom the procedure results in protracted pain despite the accurate placement of the staple line well above the dentate line. Anecdotal explanations have suggested that that this may be due to thrombosis in the residual hemorrhoidal tissue as a consequence of interruption to the hemorrhoidal venous drainage. Alternative etiologies which must be excluded include associated perianal sepsis, and acute anal fissure and sphincter spasm.

Many studies have investigated the use of adjunct therapies to reduce postoperative pain following conventional hemorrhoidectomy. These have included the use of oral metronidazole [36], agents to reduce internal sphincter spasm [37, 38], and selective use of internal sphincterotomy [39]. Few studies have been performed to investigate adjuvant therapies following stapled hemorrhoidopexy. Oral nifedipine has been reported to reduce persistent postoperative pain [40], whereas the use of oral flavinoids provides no benefit [41]. Further research is required to determine the optimal postoperative care and to maximize on the benefits of stapled hemorrhoidopexy.

Stapled Hemorrhoidopexy: Quality of Life and Cost Effectiveness

Hemorrhoidal disease is a benign condition and as such it is essential that surgical outcomes are considered in the context of quality of life (QoL). It is disappointing that so few studies have addressed this issue. Those studies that have attempted to assess QoL following stapled hemorrhoidopexy have been limited by small patient numbers, and as such it is not surprising that they have failed to show any statistically significant difference compared to conventional hemorrhoidectomy [15, 42, 43]. This goes against the intuitive feeling when one considers the quicker recovery and the general reporting of high rates of patient satisfaction following stapled hemorrhoidopexy.

Further research into QoL following stapled hemorrhoidopexy is required and should include an assessment of health resource utilization to enable a meaningful cost-effectiveness analysis to be undertaken. To date, only estimates of the in-hospital costs associated with stapled hemorrhoidopexy have been performed. Data from the NICE 2007 [16] analysis suggest that the in-hospital costs, based on the 2007 price of the stapler at £437, marginally favored conventional hemorrhoidectomy, but only by a margin of £19. If the cost of the stapler was set at the 2006 cost price of £420, then this difference diminished to only £2. The price of the PPH stapler in fact varies depending on local marketing policies and purchasing agreements. Seldom is the full-list price applicable and were this to be taken into account, together with the earlier return to normal activities and reduced use of community health care resources, it is likely that stapled hemorrhoidopexy would be superior in terms of cost effectiveness. Little information is available regarding the use of community health care resources (district nurse, general practitioner, pharmacy, etc.) following either stapled hemorrhoidopexy or conventional hemorrhoidectomy to enable an accurate cost-effective comparison. This is an area for further research and should be built into any future trials of stapled hemorrhoidopexy.

Stapled Hemorrhoidopexy and Grade of Disease

For surgeons who have accepted stapled hemorrhoidopexy the question arises as to whether or not it effectively replaces conventional excisional surgery, at least for grade III disease. It is the authors' opinion that this is unlikely to be the case. It is not an infrequent finding for patients to have isolated single pedicle prolapse. In such circumstances it is difficult to justify a full circumferential resection, the majority of which will include normal, nonprolapsing, mucohemorrhoidal tissue.

The postoperative discomfort associate with a single pedicle excision is proportionately less than that of a standard 3 pedicle excision, and probably compares favorably to stapled hemorrhoidopexy. The education of trainee surgeons in the art of conventional excisional hemorrhoidal surgery will therefore continue to be important.

There will also continue to be a need for conventional hemorrhoidectomy in acute hemorrhoidal prolapse and thrombosis. In this condition, the edematous, thrombosed piles often involve the sensitive anoderm, and it is unlikely that stapled hemorrhoidopexy will achieve satisfactory excision with an anastomosis in the required position.

A further area of controversy is whether stapled hemorrhoidopexy can be applied to all grades of prolapse (II, III, and IV) or should be restricted to grade III disease alone. Interpretation of the evidence is hindered by current classifications of hemorrhoidal disease. The Golligher classification has been used almost universally to classify disease severity in clinical studies [44]. This grading system is based on patient-reported symptoms of prolapse. The very nature of hemorrhoidal disease means that severity of symptoms will vary with the degree of prolapse present at any one time. In addition, while hemorrhoidal prolapse may be troublesome in one individual, it may be asymptomatic in another, giving a poor correlation between hemorrhoidal grade and symptomatology. An improved method of classifying hemorrhoidal disease in terms of degree of prolapse and associated symptoms is required so that surgical outcomes can be better assessed.

Accepting these limitations, evidence would suggest that stapled hemorrhoidopexy is a good option in grade III hemorrhoidal disease. Compared to other excisional techniques it offers the advantages of less pain, earlier recovery, shorter hospitalization, and perhaps less early postoperative bleeding complications. Concern remains regarding the higher rate of recurrent prolapse, and this is probably the main reason preventing its universal acceptance as the preferred technique for grade III disease.

The application of stapled hemorrhoidopexy to grade II and grade IV disease is more controversial. It is generally accepted that grade II hemorrhoidal prolapse can be adequately controlled by local treatments administered in the outpatient setting. The routine use of stapled hemorrhoidopexy in grade II prolapse cannot therefore currently be recommended, but should be reserved for patients with recurrent symptoms following failed local treatment. In grade IV prolapse, the accurate placement of the purse-string suture above the dentate line can be difficult by virtue of the volume of hemorrhoidal tissue prolapsing through the anoscope and limiting the operative view. In addition, consideration needs to be given to whether the anodermal "lift" produced by the "pexy" component of the procedure will be sufficient to deal with any external component of the prolapse, which if left untreated will manifest as residual anal skins tags which may or may not be troublesome. Stapled hemorrhoidopexy is also limited in the amount of prolapsing tissue that can be accommodated within the housing of the stapling gun, and it is all too easy to perform an inadequate excision that leaves residual prolapse. There will inevitably be some grade IV hemorrhoids in which the extent of resection required for symptomatic relief cannot be accommodated by a single PPH stapler. This may account for the higher rate of recurrent prolapse reported after stapled hemorrhoidopexy as compared to conventional hemorrhoidectomy where the extent of resection is limited only by the need to leave adequate anal skin bridges to prevent stenosis.

In the case of large grade IV prolapse the surgeon probably only has the following choices: either to revert to conventional excisional hemorrhoidectomy or if sufficiently experienced in transanal stapling techniques to consider a modified single-stapled PPH-01 resection [45] or a double-stapled PPH technique [46, 47].

It should be recognized that large hemorrhoidal prolapse is commonly accompanied by prolapse of the lower rectal mucosal, presenting as intra-anal intussusception. In these patients it has been suggested that a double-stapled PPH01 technique or STARR may be the preferred operative intervention. Boccasanta et al. randomized 64 patients with prolapsing piles and internal rectal prolapse, but no associated rectocele or enterocele, to either stapled hemorrhoidopexy or double-stapled PPH01 (STARR). The larger resection associated with the double-stapled PPH01 technique resulted in significantly less residual prolapse and a lower incidence of residual skin tags. All patients with residual disease showed prolapsed tissue over half the length of the anal dilator at the time of operation. The incidence of complications was low

in both groups, and the authors suggest that the removal of more prolapsed tissue should reduce the risk of a reintervention, justifying the higher cost of two staplers instead of one [48].

In addition to internal rectal prolapse, the surgeon planning to undertake stapled hemorrhoidopexy should be aware of the possibility of other coexistent pelvic floor abnormalities which may adversely impact on outcome. In a prospective audit of patients presenting with grade III and IV piles Schwandner et al. found that 16% had coexistent symptoms of obstructed defecation [49]. Further investigation by dynamic MRI or defecography showed additional pelvic floor pathologies in 11 of the 16 (69%) patients, of which functional disorders (dyssynergia) were the most common. As a consequence, surgical intervention was modified in all 11 patients, with eight patients undergoing biofeedback therapy, two undergoing a STARR procedure, and 1 a resectional rectopexy.

These studies underline the need for thorough preoperative evaluation and might explain some of the reported failures following stapled hemorrhoidopexy.

Stapled Transanal Rectal Resection for Obstructed Defecation Syndrome

Prior to the introduction of STARR, obstructed defecation was viewed by many as a nonsurgical entity to be treated medically by combinations of dietary modification, laxatives, and enemas. Others preferred pelvic floor retraining incorporating various forms of biofeedback therapy, or colonic lavage. If surgical correction was considered a wide range of different techniques was proposed, usually targeted at anatomical correction of a demonstrable rectocele or intussusception. The literature contains many operations aimed at the repair of rectocele and intussusception. It is not within the scope of this chapter to review all these procedures, but it is probably fair to assume that the range and number of techniques described is a reflection of their limited efficacy. Many of the operations aimed to correct an anatomical defect be it rectocele, intussusceptions, or a combination, by either suture reinforcement, rectopexy, or other pelvic floor resuspension, with or without the use of a prosthetic implant. None of these techniques dealt with the distal rectal redundancy in the same way as STARR, by full-thickness resection of the distal rectum.

The lack of a "gold standard" surgical technique for the correction of ODS hampered the initial evaluation of STARR. In the absence of an obvious comparator the design of randomized controlled trials was difficult. A dilemma therefore arose as to the best method to perform an accurate, timely assessment within a practical time-frame. Out of this dilemma emerged the concept of a prospective STARR Registry.

European STARR Registry

The introduction of STARR was a radical departure and was naturally accompanied by a degree of criticism and resistance. In addition to skepticism as to whether or not the procedure would work, there was concern regarding the potential for serious complications. In response to this, the European STARR Registry was set up in 2006. This collaboration between surgeons in Italy, the United Kingdom, and Germany aimed to rapidly accumulate data on the short-term safety and efficacy of STARR. The Registry was specifically set up with a pragmatic design. Although recommendations for inclusion and exclusion criteria were made, the final decision regarding patient selection was left to the individual surgeon. The only absolute requirement was for STARR to be performed by the double-stapled PPH-01 technique as first described by Longo. In this way, the Registry would be representative of how STARR was actually being performed in clinical practice, rather than confining it to strict pre-defined definitions and indications. An additional benefit of this approach was the facility to perform subgroup analysis on completion of the Registry, providing valuable information on the relative indications for STARR, preoperative indicators of outcome, correlation of outcomes with different surgical techniques, etc. The primary outcome measure for the STARR Registry was the change in ODS score. Secondary outcomes included change in symptom severity reporting, incontinence as assessed by the Cleveland Clinic Incontinence Score [50], and operative and postoperative complications. In addition, quality of life was assessed using the symptom-specific Patient Assessment of Constipation (PAC-QoL) [51] and the generic EQ-5D [52] questionnaires. Data were collected preoperatively, and at 6 weeks and 6 and 12 months postoperatively into a centralized, anonymous database. Data monitoring was the responsibility of each individual country, performed under the auspices of its national coloproctological society.

Within 12 months, the Registry had amassed data on over 1,500 patients. Analysis of the 12-month follow-up data has shown a significant improvement in the ODS and symptom severity scores (Fig. 9.1)

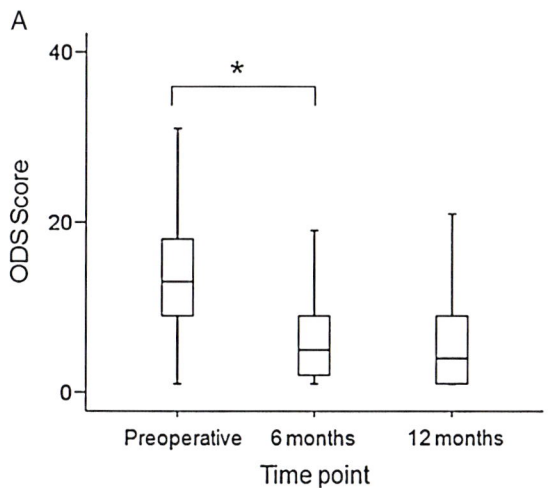
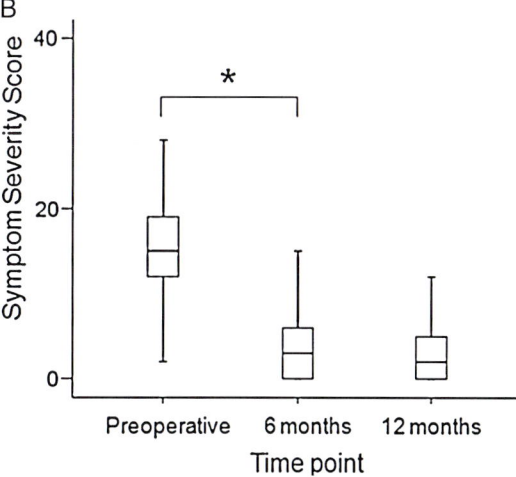

Fig. 9.1. Comparison of ODS and SSS scores at preoperative, 6- and 12-month follow-up. A significant improvement in both ODS (**a**) and SSS (**b**) was observed between baseline and 6 months, which was maintained at 12 months. *Paired t test, $P < 0.001$

as well as the PAC-QoL and ED-5Q quality-of-life assessments (Figs. 9.2 and 9.3) following STARR. The overall morbidity, including all minor and major complications, was acceptable at 32% with the most common complications being defecatory urgency (16.2%), urinary retention (6.3%), and bleeding (4.3%) (Table 9.1). One serious septic complication due to necrosis at the stapled anastomosis was reported which required the formation of a defunctioning stoma. One rectovaginal fistula occurred. There was no reported mortality.

Incontinence is always a concern with any transanal surgery, and this is particularly so following STARR. A change in continence is, however, difficult to assess objectively following STARR as it is frequently a component of the ODS symptom complex prior to any surgical intervention. Thus, 11.2% of patients had a Cleveland Clinic incontinence score of ≥ 3 preoperatively. This compared to 8% and 5.1% with an incontinence score of ≥ 3 at 6- and 12 months postoperatively, respectively (Fig. 9.4). Thus, as a group an overall

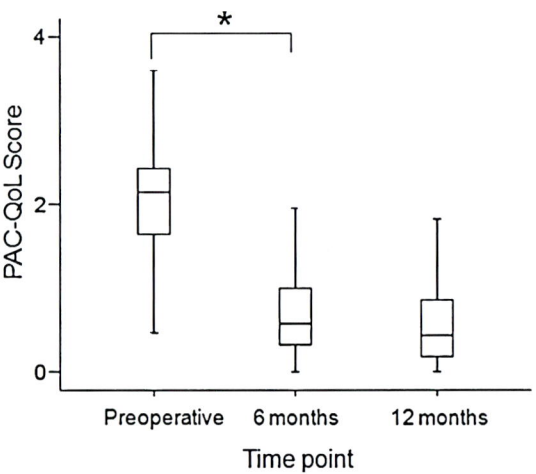

FIG. 9.2. Comparison of PAQ-QOL scores at preoperative, 6- and 12-month follow-up. A significant improvement was observed between baseline and 6 months, which was maintained at 12 months. *Paired t test, $p < 0.001$

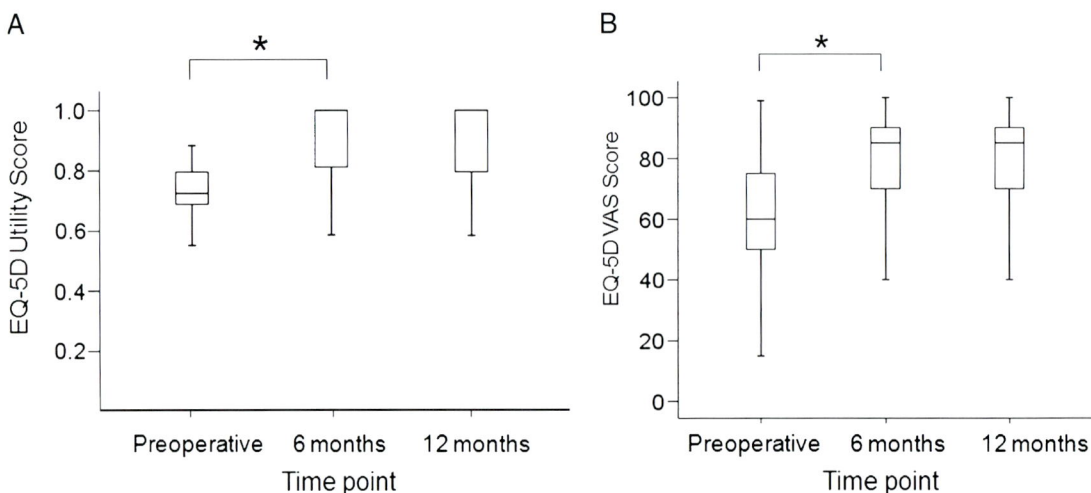

FIG. 9.3. Comparison of EQ-5D scores at preoperative, 6- and 12-month follow-up. A significant improvement was observed in both the Utility Score (**a**) and the Visual Analogue Score (**b**) between baseline and 6 months, which was maintained at 12 months. *Paired t test, $p < 0.001$

Table 9.1. Combined reporting of complications (operative, perioperative, and postoperative) in 2,638 patients entered into Registry.

Complication	N (%)
Defecatory urgency	427 (16.2)
Urinary retention	165 (6.3)
Bleeding	109 (4.1)
Stapled line complication	76 (2.9)
Sepsis	36 (1.4)
Incontinence	34 (1.3)
Anastomotic stenosis	4 (0.5)
Dysperunia	2 (0.1)
Rectal necrosis	1 (0.04)
Rectovaginal fistula	1 (0.04)
Mortality	0 (0)

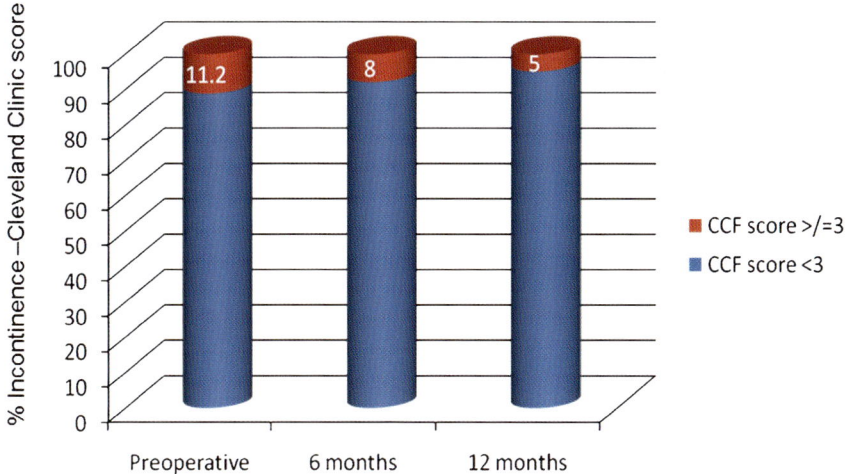

Fig. 9.4. Comparison of the symptom "incontinence" as determined by a Cleveland Clinic Score ≥ 3 at preoperative, 6- and 12-month follow-up. Incontinence is a feature of the preoperative ODS symptom complex which improves with time following STARR

significant improvement in incontinence symptoms as observed (preoperative mean = 0.85, 95%CI: 0.74–0.96; 6 months' mean = 0.59, 95%CI: 0.40–0.60; 12 months' mean = 0.40, 95%CI: 0.32–0.49; $p < 0.001$). This was mirrored by a significant improvement in patient-reported symptoms of incontinence/soiling which was a component of the Symptom Severity Score. It would therefore appear that there is an overall improvement in incontinent symptoms, which is most marked at 12-months follow-up. However, a minority of patients will experience a worsening of incontinence, and this is probably reflected in the 1.3% incontinence rate reported as a complication of the procedure (Table 9.1).

A similar argument holds true for defecatory urgency. Although this is frequently reported as a complication of the STARR procedure it is also a feature of the preoperative ODS symptom complex. Thus, the 16.2% defecatory urgency rate reported at 12 months following STARR is unlikely to be the true incidence of *de novo* urgency. The only tool available in the Registry to analyze defecatory urgency was the Symptom Severity Score. One component of this score recorded "difficulty to withstand urge to open bowels" on a 5-point scale (0 = none of the time, 1 = a little of the time, 2 = some of the time, 3 = most of the time, 4 = all the time). Analysis of this data showed that defecatory urgency was experienced "most of the time" or "all

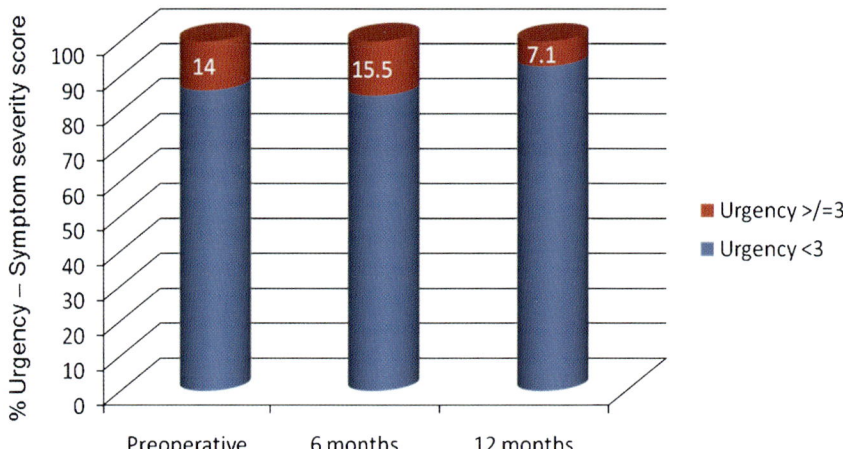

F<small>IG</small>. 9.5. Comparison of the symptom "defecatory urgency" as determined by a symptom severity score ≥ 3 at preoperative, 6- and 12- month follow-up. Urgency is a feature of the preoperative ODS symptom complex which improves with time following STARR

the time" (score ≥ 3) in 14% of patients preoperatively, and in 15.5% and 7.1% of patients at 6- and 12-months follow-up, respectively. Thus, it would appear that as a group there was an improvement in defecatory urgency following STARR, which was most marked at the 12 month follow-up time point (Fig. 9.5).

The STARR Registry was set up specifically to provide a rapid audit of the safety and efficacy of STARR prior to its widespread dissemination. As such, it is likely to achieve its purpose. However, as a prospective audit it has its limitations, with voluntary participation and a pragmatic design making it susceptible to biases in patient selection and the reporting of complications. Specifically designed randomized trials are now required.

Future Assessment of STARR by Randomized Comparison

Further assessment of STARR in randomized controlled trials is required, but the problem remains as to the choice of a suitable comparator. No "gold standard" surgical treatment for obstructed defecation exists. Rectocele repair, whether performed by the transanal, transvaginal, or perineal approach, is nonresectional and as such does not address the distal rectal redundancy and prolapse in the same way as STARR. Similarly, conventional rectopexy

procedures for intussusception or internal prolapse are associated with poor results in terms of correction of rectal evacuatory function. Recently, there has been renewed interest in ventral rectopexy procedures for the treatment of rectal prolapse and intussusception, but the outcome data to date remain limited [53, 54]. Probably the best comparator is the "internal" Delorme's procedure, but this can be a difficult and bloody procedure that is unlikely to be accepted as a technical equivalent by the majority of surgeons.

Evaluation of outcome data from clinical trials is also hampered by the lack of a validated measure of obstructed defecation. The Obstructed Defecation Score proposed by Longo has been accepted and used in clinical trials without formal evaluation. Although it is valuable in comparing symptoms before and after STARR, and as a comparator of case mix in different clinical studies, it suffers from several weaknesses. It is derived by summation of nine component scores. Some of these components are assessed in a subjective manner making it vulnerable to patient interpretation and interobserver variation. There has been no correlation between ODS score and its impact on quality of life: a high ODS score in one individual may indicate significant symptomatology, whereas in another it may be accepted as normal. It has been variously suggested that an ODS score > 7 or > 9 represents pathological disease and should be an indication for STARR.

But the ODS score is merely an attempt to quantify a patient's symptoms of evacuatory dysfunction and should not be used as an indicator for surgical intervention or a predictor of outcome. It has been estimated that some 14% of "normal" women will exhibit an ODS score > 9 in the absence of symptoms necessitating surgical intervention [55].

Although various modifications of the original ODS scoring system have been proposed only that proposed by Altomare et al. has been evaluated and then only in an Italian population [56]. This scoring system bears a close resemblance to that proposed by Longo but has the advantage that all component scores are categorized. For practical purposes, it would be desirable to see this or another validated scoring system adopted as the international standard to facilitate data interpretation and future research.

The early evidence with STARR suggests that it is an effective treatment for ODS associated with an anatomical redundancy of the distal rectum. This includes patients with rectoceles associated with ODS. There therefore arises the contentious issue as to which specialty of surgeon, the coloproctologist or the gynecologist, is best equipped to treat the condition. Should the gynecologist perform a rectocele repair in the hope that it will lead to a secondary improvement in rectal evacuation, or should the coloproctologist perform a STARR procedure, which is primarily aimed at treating rectal dysfunction, with secondary correction of the rectocele? In the United Kingdom at least, the majority of rectocele repairs are performed by gynecologists. It remains unknown how many of these patients also have rectal evacuatory dysfunction, and it is unlikely that bowel symptoms are adequately assessed as part of the work-up for gynecological surgery. Although the presence of a rectocele *per se* is not an indication for operative intervention, being present in asymptomatic females [57, 58], those patients presenting with a symptomatic rectocele should at least be screened for coexistent defecatory dysfunction. A gynecological approach to rectocele repair seems justified if symptoms are vaginal in nature (protrusion per vagina or dysperunia) in the absence of obstructive defecation symptoms. However, if rectal evacuatory symptoms coexist then appropriate preoperative investigation should include defecating proctography or dynamic MRI to identify any internal rectal prolapse, which might be correctable by STARR. A randomized clinical trial comparing transvaginal rectocele repair with STARR in patients with symptoms of ODS would help to clarify this area of uncertainty.

Controversies Specific to STARR

The optimal preoperative work-up for patients with ODS prior to operative selection remains unknown. There can be little argument that some form of dynamic radiological imaging of pelvic floor is required, either by conventional contrast proctography or dynamic MRI (see Chap. 4). However, the indications for anorectal physiology, endoanal ultrasound, and colonic transit studies remain unclear.

The effect of coexistent slow transit constipation on the outcome of STARR is yet to be determined. Conversely, circumstantial evidence suggests that removing the distal obstructive component may have a beneficial effect on overall colonic motility.

Provided the patient has good sphincter tone and squeeze on digital examination and there is no history of fecal incontinence, it is probably reasonable to omit formal sphincter evaluation. The difficulty comes in those patients with a potentially compromised anal sphincter who will be at particular risk of defecatory urgency and incontinence following STARR. In these patients, preoperative anorectal physiology testing and endoanal ultrasound are probably mandatory in order to properly advise the patient.

Patients with ODS and poor anal sphincter function are likely to present a mixed picture of evacuatory obstruction combined with urgency and incontinence. It can often be difficult to distinguish whether urgency and incontinence is a feature of the ODS or a function of poor sphincter control. In these complex patients a tailored approach, supported by anorectal physiology data, and based on the predominant symptom is advised. If the predominant symptom is obstructed defecation, it might be reasonable to recommend STARR as the initial intervention with the caveat that it might result in unacceptable urgency or even incontinence, requiring a second intervention either in the form of sphincter repair or augmentation with sacral nerve stimulation. In patients where incontinence is the predominant symptom, repair of a sphincter defect is probably not recommended in the first instance as it is likely to exacerbate any obstructive symptoms, which will not then be amenable to a subsequent STARR procedure for fear of disrupting the repaired sphincter. Similarly, it is probably ill-advised to perform STARR as the initial intervention as it is likely to worsen incontinence, although it could be argued that once the obstructive element has been corrected the incontinence may be controllable with constipating agents.

The male patient with ODS presents a challenging proposition. The etiology underlying male evacuatory dysfunction is less well characterized and is likely to be different to that observed in the female. Provided internal rectal prolapse can be demonstrated on dynamic radiological imaging, it is reasonable to advocate STARR for males with ODS provided the patient is aware that there are no published data to support its efficacy and that any evidence for success is drawn by extrapolation from the female on the basis of correction of an anatomical abnormality. To date, a limited number of male patients with ODS symptoms have been treated with STARR and entered into the European Registry. Preliminary results would suggest that there is a benefit in symptom improvement. However, the anatomy of the male pelvis dictates that on average the degree of internal intussusception is likely to be less than in the female, and for this reason the double-stapled PPH01 technique is preferred to the Contour30 (Transtar); the Contour30 being technically more difficult for small internal prolapse.

The optimal management of patients with obstructed defecation secondary to functional rather than anatomical anomalies of the pelvic floor is yet to be clearly defined. Functional pelvic floor problems comprise a group of disorders variously referred to as anismus, puborectalis paradoxus, pelvic dyssynergia, and spastic pelvic floor syndrome. The diagnosis, let alone the treatment of these disorders, remains controversial. STARR cannot be recommended for these disorders when they exist in the absence of a demonstrable anatomical defect. However, greater experience will determine the benefit or otherwise of STARR when there is coexistent internal prolapse. Currently, the best form of therapy for these patients is probably a combination of best medical management in conjunction with biofeedback or colonic irrigation. The potential role of sacral nerve modulation in these patients remains to be clarified.

Patients with solitary rectal ulcer syndrome (SRUS) are another interesting group. It is well recognized that in a proportion of these patients there will have an internal prolapse demonstrable on dynamic imaging. Hypothetically, STARR should offer a benefit in these patients, but to date evidence remains anecdotal. Typically, a solitary rectal ulcer is situated on the anterior rectal wall at 7–8 cm from the anal verge. It would appear ill-advised to offer STARR in the presence of active ulceration, when the tissues will be edematous with tethering of the ulcerated rectum to the rectovaginal septum. However, if active ulceration can be temporarily resolved by aggressive medical management then it may be reasonable to offer STARR to remove the offending internal prolapse and prevent symptom recurrence.

Internal rectal prolapse is frequently accompanied by prolapse of the anterior and middle pelvic compartments, requiring multidisciplinary investigation and intervention. The presence of multicompartment prolapse suggests a common underlying etiology related to stretching and weakness of the endopelvic fascia with or without pelvic neuropathy. Dynamic MRI is likely to be most beneficial in such patients, helping to identify the predominant anatomical abnormality and guiding surgical treatment. For example, marked uterine prolapse may be sufficient to explain coexisting rectal evacuatory dysfunction, with hysterectomy alone being sufficient treatment. STARR can then be reserved for patients with persistent ODS symptoms which have failed to respond to hysterectomy. In other instances, internal rectal and uterine prolapse may coexist in equal proportion, such that hysterectomy and STARR are best performed at the same operation. Such patients present a formidable diagnostic and therapeutic challenge and should be treated within the context of a dedicated multidisciplinary pelvic floor clinic.

Postoperative defecatory urgency is variously reported in 10–30% of patients following the STARR procedure. This has been the focus for criticism by some authorities [59]. However, what the literature often fails to report is the existence of preoperative defecatory urgency which is a recognized feature of ODS. If this is taken into account the incidence of *de novo* postoperative urgency is much reduced, and preoperative urgency is actually improved for many patients. Although urgency usually improves during the first 3–6 months postoperatively there are a small proportion of patients in whom it remains problematic. It is probable that these patients had a weakened anal sphincter preoperatively, a tendency to loose bowel habit, or irritable bowel syndrome that was not fully appreciated on preoperative assessment. Identifying such patients by appropriate use of preoperative anorectal physiology is essential, as the occurrence of intractable defecatory urgency is a difficult clinical problem to manage.

The last decade has seen a renewed interest in the treatment of pelvic floor dysfunction. This has been driven in part by the introduction of stapled hemorrhoidopexy and STARR, by the development of meshes for gynecological pelvic floor repair, and by the potential benefits of sacral nerve modulation. It has yet to be determined where STARR fits into the algorithm of multicompartment pelvic floor failure. The favorable results of sacral nerve modulation for the treatment of fecal incontinence has led several researchers to explore the possibility of this modality as an option for constipation-related disorders with some degree of success [60, 61]. Sacral nerve modulation may be particularly applicable in those cases of mixed defecatory dysfunction where constipation symptoms coexist with weakened anal sphincter function putting the patient at an unacceptable risk of intractable defecatory urgency should they be subjected to STARR. A randomized trial of STARR vs. sacral nerve modulation for mixed defecatory dysfunction would provide useful information.

Double-Stapled PPH01 or Contour30 (Transtar) for ODS?

Longo's initial description of the STARR procedure involved the use of a double-stapling technique with the PPH01 device, a stapler that had been designed for the treatment of prolapsing piles rather than full-thickness rectal resection. Although the double-stapled PPH technique has been proven to be effective, at least in the short term, it has its limitations. Circumferential resection is performed in two stages: an anterior and a posterior resection.

This can result in an inadequate resection in the area where the anterior and posterior resections meet, with the formation of lateral "dog-ears." The resection is performed in a semi-blinded fashion; the traction sutures are inserted and used to pull the prolapsing rectum into the stapler housing with little scope for operator control of the extent of the resection performed. In addition, the extent of the resection is restricted to the amount of tissue that can be accommodated within the stapler housing, limiting the ability to resect a large prolapse.

The Contour30 (Transtar) was designed specifically to overcome some of the technical difficulties associated with the double-stapled PPH01 STARR. The reader is referred to Chap. 7 for details of the instrument and operative technique. With the Contour30 the operator is afforded greater control over the operation in terms of the extent of prolapse to be resected, which can be tailored to the individual patient. The resection can be performed under direct vision and a uniform full-thickness circumferential resection achieved without the lateral "dog-ears" seen after double-stapled PPH resection. If required, a greater volume of tissue can be incorporated into the Contour30 device ensuring complete resection of a large prolapse. Initial experience with the Contour30 would suggest that it is as safe and effective as the double-stapled PPH01 technique. Whether the ability to resect larger volumes of rectal prolapse translates into an improvement in outcomes remains to be seen.

Currently, there therefore exist two staplers and two techniques for performing STARR. Whether the Contour30 (Transtar) will eventually replace the double-stapled PPH01 technique completely is unknown. The two techniques are not necessarily interchangeable, and it may be that each technique has its own indications within the context of anorectal prolapse. It is likely that the majority of patients with ODS will be suitable for Contour30 (Transtar) resection, which in moderate-to-large prolapses will produce a superior volume of resection. However, in patients with a small prolapse (in the region of 2 cm or less) the Contour30 can be a difficult procedure and the double-stapled PHH01 technique may continue to be the preferred option. For reasons discussed earlier, the double-stapled PPH01 technique may also remain the procedure of choice in the male patient and the patient with large volume hemorrhoids and associated rectal mucosal prolapse, where the volume of tissue to be resected cannot be adequately accommodated by a single firing of the PPH01 or PPH03 stapler. For the immediate future the coloproctologist will continue to have both staplers (PPH01 and Contour30) and both techniques at his disposable and until such time as appropriate randomized trials are performed should exercise judgment on an individual patient basis as to the best way to proceed.

Summary

Over the last decade transanal stapling has established itself as a credible alternative for the treatment of anorectal prolapse. Stapled hemorrhoidopexy has been subjected to evaluation in many randomized controlled trials and meta-analyses and has proven early benefits in terms of reduced postoperative pain, shorter hospital stay, and earlier return to normal function. Continuing controversies prevent it from being universally accepted. Previous concerns regarding early postoperative complications have largely been resolved and appear to be related to surgical technique. There remains the continuing issue of higher rates of recurrent prolapse on long-term follow-up, which may be due to an inability of the stapler to accommodate large prolapsing piles. In patients with prolapsing piles and associated rectal mucosal prolapse stapled hemorrhoidopexy is unlikely to achieve an adequate resection. This has been addressed by modifications of the original PPH technique including the use of a double-stapled PPH01 STARR procedure. Further evaluation of the quality of life and cost effectiveness associated with stapled hemorrhoidopexy is required.

The introduction of the STARR procedure promises to revolutionize the treatment of ODS associated with internal rectal prolapse. Preliminary results have been encouraging, but long-term follow-up data are required. Like any new technique uncertainties remain regarding the indications for STARR, particularly when ODS coexists in the presence of slow transit constipation, irritable bowel syndrome, and other functional pelvic floor disorders. Currently, two staplers and two techniques are available for STARR. Whether the greater resection afforded by the Contour 30 stapler translates into better clinical outcomes remains to be seen.

An emerging concept proposes that internal rectal prolapse and prolapsing hemorrhoids share a common etiology. This provides an interesting area for further investigations and may come to influence our future understanding and treatment of anorectal prolapse disease.

References

1. Longo A: Treatment of haemorrhoidal disease by reduction of mucosal and haemorrhoidal prolapse with a circular stapling device: a new procedure. Proceedings of the sixth World Congress of Endoscopic Surgery. Rome, Italy, 1998
2. Rowsell M, Bello M, Hemingway DM: Circumferential mucosectomy (stapled haemorrhoidectomy) versus conventional haemorrhoidectomy: randomised controlled trial. Lancet 2000; 355:779–781
3. Mehigan BJ, Monson JR, Hartely JE: Stapling procedure for haemorrhoids versus Milligan–Morgan haemorrhoidectomy: randomised controlled trial. Lancet 2000; 355: 782–785
4. Cheetham MJ, Mortensen NJ, Nystrom PO, Kamm MA, Phillips RK: Persistent pain and faecal urgency after stapled haemorrhoidectomy. Lancet 2000; 356: 730–733
5. Pescatori M: Pain after stapled haemorrhoidectomy. Lancet 2000; 356: 2188
6. Molloy RG, Kingsmore D: Life threatening pelvic sepsis after stapled haemorrhoidectomy. Lancet 2000; 355: 810
7. Shalaby R, Desoky A: Randomized clinical trial of stapled versus Milligan–Morgan haemorrhoidectomy. Br J Surg 2001; 88: 1049–1053
8. Ho YH, Cheong WK, Tsang C, Ho J, Eu KW, Tang CL, Seow-Choen F: Stapled hemorrhoidectomy – cost and effectiveness. Randomized, controlled trial including incontinence scoring, anorectal manometry, and endoanal ultrasound assessments at up to three months. Dis Colon Rectum 2000; 43: 1666–1675
9. Senagore AJ, Singer M, Abcarian H, Fleshman J, Corman M, Wexner S, Nivatvongs S: Procedure for Prolapse and Hemorrhoids (PPH) Multicenter Study Group: A prospective, randomized, controlled multicenter trial comparing stapled hemorrhoidopexy and Ferguson hemorrhoidectomy: perioperative and one-year results. Dis Colon Rectum 2004; 47: 1824–1836
10. Boccasanta P, Capretti PG, VM: Randomised controlled trial between stapled circumferential mucosectomy and conventional circular hemorrhoidectomy in advanced hemorrhoids with external mucosal prolapse. Am J Surg 2001; 182: 64–68

11. Pavlidis T, Papaziogas B, Souparis A: Modern stapled Longo procedure vs. conventional Milligan–Morgan hemorrhoidectomy: a randomized controlled trial. Int J Colorectal Dis 2002; 17: 50–53

12. Correa-Rovelo JM, Tellez O, Obregan L: Stapled rectal mucosectomy vs. closed hemorrhoidectomy: a randomized, clinical trial. Dis Colon Rectum 2002; 45: 1367–1374

13. Ortiz H, Marzo J, Armendariz P: Randomized clinical trial of stapled haemorrhoidopexy versus conventional diathermy haemorrhoidectomy. Br J Surg 2002; 89: 1376–1381

14. Ganio E, Altomare DF, Gabrielli F, Milito G, Canuti S: Prospective randomized multicentre trial comparing stapled with open haemorrhoidectomy. Br J Surg 2001; 88: 669–674

15. Smyth EF, Baker RP, Wilken BJ, Hartley JE, White TJ, Monson JR: Stapled versus excision haemorrhoidectomy: long-term follow up of a randomised controlled trial. Lancet 2003; 361: 1437–1438

17. Nisar P.J, Acheson A.G, Neal K.R, Scholefield J.H: Stapled hemorrhoidopexy compared with conventional hemorrhoidectomy: systematic review of randomized controlled trials. Dis Colon Rectum 2004; 47: 1837–1845

19. Brusciano L, Ayabaca SM, Pescatori M, Accarpio GM, Dodi G, Cavallari F, Ravo B, Annibali R: Reinterventions after complicated or failed stapled hemorrhoidopexy. Dis Colon Rectum 2004; 47: 1846–1851

20. Finco C, Sarzo G, Savastano S, Degregori S, Merigliano S: Stapled haemorrhoidopexy in fourth degree haemorrhoidal prolapse: is it worthwhile? Colorectal Dis 2006; 8: 130–134

21. Nisar PJ, Acheson AG, Neal KR, Scholefield JH: Stapled hemorrhoidopexy compared with conventional hemorrhoidectomy: systematic review of randomized, controlled trials. Dis Colon Rectum 2004; 47: 1837–1845

22. Oughriss M, Yver R, Faucheron JL: Complications of stapled hemorrhoidectomy: a French multicentric study. Gastroenterologie Clinique et Biologique 2005; 29: 429–433

23. Ravo B, Amato A, Bianco V, Boccasanta P, Bottini C, Carriero A, Milito G, Dodi G, Mascagni D, Orsini S, Pietroletti R, Ripetti V, Tagariello GB: Complications after stapled hemorrhoidectomy: can they be prevented? Tech Coloproctol 2002; 6: 83–88

24. Tjandra JJ, Chan MK: Systematic review on the procedure for prolapse and hemorrhoids (stapled hemorrhoidopexy). Dise Colon Rectum 2007; 50: 878–892

25. Van de SJ, D'Hoore A, Duinslaeger M, Chasse E, Penninckx F: Belgian Section of Colorectal Surgery Royal Belgian Society for Surgery: Long-term results after excision haemorrhoidectomy versus stapled haemorrhoidopexy for prolapsing haemorrhoids; a Belgian prospective randomized trial. Acta Chirurgica Belgica 2005; 105: 44–52

26. Fueglistaler P, Guenin MO, Montali I, Kern B, Peterli R, von FM, Ackermann C: Long-term results after stapled hemorrhoidopexy: high patient satisfaction despite frequent postoperative symptoms. Dis Colon Rectum 2007; 50: 204–212

27. Guenin MO, Rosenthal R, Kern B, Peterli R, von FM, Ackermann C: Ferguson hemorrhoidectomy: long-term results and patient satisfaction after Ferguson's hemorrhoidectomy. Dis Colon Rectum 2005; 48: 1523–1527

28. Peng BC, Jayne DG, Ho YH: Randomized trial of rubber band ligation vs. stapled hemorrhoidectomy for prolapsed piles. Dis Colon Rectum 2003; 46: 291–297

29. Shanmugam V, Watson AJ, Chapman AD, Binnie NR, Loudon MA: Pathological audit of stapled haemorrhoidopexy. Colorectal Dis 2005; 7: 172–175

30. Plocek MD, Kondylis LA, Duhan-Floyd N, Reilly JC, Geisler DP, Kondylis PD: Hemorrhoidopexy staple line height predicts return to work. Dis Colon Rectum 2006; 49: 1905–1909

31. Williams R, Kondylis L, Geisler D, Kondylis P: Stapled hemorrhoidopexy height as outcome indicator. Am J Surg 2007; 193: 336–339

32. Arroyo A, Perez-Vicente F, Miranda E, Sanchez A, Serrano P, Candela F, Oliver I, Calpena R: Prospective randomized clinical trial comparing two different circular staplers for mucosectomy in the treatment of hemorrhoids. World J Surg 2006; 30: 1305–1310

33. Esser S, Khubchandani I, Rakhmanine M: Stapled hemorrhoidectomy with local anesthesia can be performed safely and cost-efficiently. Dis Colon Rectum 2004; 47: 1164–1169

34. Ong CH, Chee Boon FE, Keng V: Ambulatory circular stapled haemorrhoidectomy under local anaesthesia versus circular stapled haemorrhoidectomy under regional anaesthesia. ANZ J Surg 2005; 75: 184–186

35. Law WL, Tung HM, Chu KW, Lee FC: Ambulatory stapled haemorrhoidectomy: a safe and feasible surgical technique. Hong Kong Med J 2003; 9: 103–107

36. Carapeti EA, Kamm MA, McDonald PJ, Phillips RK: Double-blind randomised controlled trial of effect of metronidazole on pain after day-case haemorrhoidectomy. Lancet 1998; 351: 169–172

37. Tan KY, Sng KK, Tay KH, Lai JH, Eu KW: Randomized clinical trial of 0.2 per cent glyceryl trinitrate ointment for wound healing and pain reduction after open diathermy haemorrhoidectomy. Br J Surg 2006; 93: 1464–1468

38. Patti R, Angileri M, Migliore G, Sammartano S, Termine S, Crivello F, Gioe FP, Di VG: Effectiveness of contemporary injection of botulinum toxin and topical application of glyceryl trinitrate against postoperative pain after Milligan–Morgan haemorrhoidectomy. Annali Italiani di Chirurgia 2006; 77: 503–508

39. Mathai V, Ong BC, Ho YH: Randomized controlled trial of lateral internal sphincterotomy with haemorrhoidectomy. Br J Surg 1996; 83: 380–382

40. Thaha MA, Irvine LA, Steele RJ, Campbell KL: Postdefaecation pain syndrome after circular stapled anopexy is abolished by oral nifedipine. Br J Surg 2005; 92: 208–210

41. Mlakar B, Kosorok P: Flavonoids to reduce bleeding and pain after stapled hemorrhoidopexy: a randomized controlled trial. Wiener Klinische Wochenschrift 2005; 117: 558–560

42. Wilson MS, Pope V, Doran HE, Fearn SJ, Brough WA: Objective comparison of stapled anopexy and open hemorrhoidectomy: a randomized, controlled trial. Dis Colon Rectum 2002; 45: 1437–1444

43. Mehigan BJ, Monson JR, Hartley JE: Stapling procedure for haemorrhoids versus Milligan–Morgan haemorrhoidectomy: randomised controlled trial. Lancet 2000; 355: 782–785

44. Goligher JC: Surgery of the anus, rectum and colon. ed 5th ed., London, Bailliere Tindall, 1984

45. Jayne DG, Seow-Choen F: Modified stapled haemorrhoidopexy for the treatment of massive circumferentially prolapsing piles. Tech Coloproctol 2002; 6: 191–193

46. Boccasanta P, Venturi M, Gaincario R: Stapled transanal rectal resection versus stapled anopexy in the cure of hemorrhoids associated with rectal prolapse. A randomised controlled trial. Int J Colorectal Dis 2007; 22: 245–251

47. Papagrigoriadis S, Vardonikolaki A: Stapled anopexy with double stapling: a safe and efficient treatment for fourth degree haemorrhoids. Acta Chirurgica Belgica 2006; 106: 717–718

48. Slawik S, Kenefick N, Greenslade GL, Dixon AR: A prospective evaluation of stapled haemorrhoidopexy/rectal mucosectomy in the management of 3rd and 4th degree haemorrhoids. Colorectal Dis 2007; 9: 352–356

49. Schwandner O, Bruch HP: Significance of obstructed defaecation in haemorrhoidal disease: results of a prospective study. Coloproctol 2006; 28: 13–20

50. Jorge JM, Wexner SD: Etiology and management of fecal incontinence. Dis Colon Rectum 1993; 36: 77–97

51. Marquist P, De La Loge C, Dubois D, McDermott A, Chassaney O: Development and validation of the Patient Assessment of Constipation Quality of Life questionnaire. Scand J Gastroenterol 2005; 40: 540–551

52. Brooks P: EuroQol: the current state of play. Health Policy 1996; 37: 53–72

53. Portier G, Iovino F, Lazorthes F: Surgery for rectal prolapse: Orr-Loygue ventral rectopexy with limited dissection prevents postoperative-induced constipation without increasing recurrence. Dis Colon Rectum 2006; 49: 1136–1140

54. D'Hoore A, Cadoni R, Penninckx F: Long-term outcome of laparoscopic ventral rectopexy for total rectal prolapse. Br J Surgery 2004; 91: 1500–1505

55. Mockford K, Loughenbury P, Culverwell A, Jayne DG: Ob-structed defecation syndrome: a comparism of the ODS and KESS scoring systems. 2nd World Congress of coloproctology and pelvic disease, 2007. Rome

56. Altomore DF, Spazzafuma L, Rinaldi M, Dodi G, Ghiselli R, Piloni V: Set-up and statistical validation of a new scoring system for obstructed defaecation syndrome. Colorectal Dis 2008; 10: 84–88

57. Bartram CJ, Turnball GK, Lennard-Jones JE: Evacuation proctography, an investigation of rectal expulsion in twenty subjects without defecatory disturbance. Gastrointest Radiol 1988; 13: 72–80

58. Shorovan PJ, McHugh S, Diamant NE, Somers S, Stevenson GW: Defecography in normal volunteers, results and implications. Gut 1989; 30: 1737–1749

59. Dodi G, Pietroletti R, Milito G, Binda G, Pescatori M: Bleeding, incontinence, pain and constipation after STARR transanal double stapling rectotomy for obstructed defecation. Tech Coloproctology 2003; 7: 148–153

60. Ganio F, Masin A, Ratto C, Altomore DF, Ripetti V, Clerico G, Lise M, Daglietto GB, Memeo V, landolfi V, Del Genio A, Arullani A, Giardiello G, ds Seta F: Short-term sacral nerve stimulation for functional anorectal and urinary disturbances: results in 40 patients. Dis Colon Rectum 2002; 44: 1261–1267

61. Kenefick NJ, Vaizey CJ, Cohen CRG, Nicholls CJ, Kamm MA: Double-blind placebo-controlled crossover study of sacral nerve stimulation for idiopathic constipation. Br J Surg 2002; 89: 1570–1571

Index